THE SECRET
Whom Does It Protect?

*My sister and I
were too young to have had such a
a frightening experience.*

The Screams, And The Cover-Up.

BY:JAY FOSTER

THE SECRET
Copyright © 2021 by Jay Foster

No part of this non-fiction publication may be copied, reproduced in any format, by any means, electronic or otherwise, without prior consent from the copyright owner and publisher of this book.

Dedication

To my father, Kenneth,
You were the greatest single dad I know.
The life lessons that you taught me, I passed on to my kids.
I will always have you in my heart.

Acknowledgments

I must give special acknowledgment and recognition to my three brilliant children: To my son Chris, and my daughters, Jo and Toni, for their love, inspiration, advice, and for all their help and support as I build up the courage to tell my story and finally free myself from the prison this secret had me locked in for decades.

I must also recognize and acknowledge the family I grew up in for its support and encouragement throughout the years: My sister Celia, may she RIP... Yvonne, Angie, Janet, Maureen, and my brother Winston. I will also use this time to acknowledge my Mother Ivy, my half-brothers Paul, may his soul RIP... Garry and Barry.

I am also grateful to my many friends for their love and support. Thanks to Tarans Burke for creating #MeToo, which has become a movement. You have afforded me a non-judgmental platform to state my truth without being evaluated.

Thank you to all the courageous women and men who shared their stories of sexual assault. I must say, your courage has given me the power to tell my story—those of you who are still afraid to talk about the unwanted sexual advances you experienced. I am here to tell you that the current climate gives you the security and support you require when you're trying to get rid of the shame and guilt that's been haunting you for years—talking about what happened to me has liberated me.

Foreword

We Cried Together, and Then We Kept Quiet!

My sister and I kept an enormous childhood secret from the world because we were scared of what people would think and say about us. We kept the secret locked away to the point of never discussing it with ourselves nor our family.

When the #MeToo movement began, however, I finally decided to bring my traumatic story to the forefront, sharing thoroughly with the world what happened to us that day many years ago. After having to hold on to so many unexpressed emotions for so long, I decided to free myself by giving a detail-oriented synapse of my life, providing insights into a journey that has taken years to overcome. The #MeToo movement has changed the culture surrounding all unwanted sexual advances. It gave me the freedom, courage, and unwavering inspiration to speak my truth about the sexual misconduct my sister and I encountered without the fear of being judged.

This movement serves as a platform that sheds light on the many untold stories, giving a voice to many women and men hiding in the shadows, suppressed by heavy guilt and melancholy. These persons no longer feel alone as this movement empowers every corner of their souls. We finally have the opportunity to speak of our suffering without cowering in the shame and guilt often experienced by victims of sexual harassment, rape, and sexual assault. Now the door is wide open for all those who have suffered at the hands of insensitive, despicable, malicious persons to speak out without feeling blamed or fearful.

On shifting the stigma from the victim's humiliation to the perpetrator's inhumanities, I realized that I had to seize this crucial moment to talk about what had happened to me. If I didn't have the guts to speak now, vocalizing the cruelty that stained my childhood, I probably would never get another chance. And maybe I would have to hold my peace forever, never knowing if my story had influenced someone out there who, as I had, felt too afraid to speak.

In all honesty, I can say that I give full credit to the #MeToo movement for giving me a platform to tell my story without fear. It has helped motivate me tremendously in breaking my silence after holding onto it for so many years. Hence, I have to admit that without it, I would probably have died without being able to rid myself of the shame and guilt an inhumane act had inflicted on me. Bearing such a silence, my kids would never, for a second, fathom how their lives were affected by my rape experience.

Table of Contents

Dedication 3
Acknowledgments 4
Foreword 6
Introduction 1
The #MeToo Freed Me from My Shame 11
I Cried for Her, and Then I Cried for Me 21
The Day My Life Changed Paths 28
Questions for the Rapists 37
How Your Actions Affected My Psyche 45
The Shame, Guilt and Blame 49
How the Rape Affected My Parenting 66
It Was Called Battery 80
The Rapists' Reputation 84
How It Affected My Well-being 94
How I Will Tell My Children 105
How I Freed Myself from the Secret 108
Writing This Book Helped Me 114
Thank You Ladies and Gentlemen 132
Raising Compassionate Men Can Teach Empathy ... 135
Teach Random Acts of Kindness - Teach Compassion ... 143

Introduction

Sexual assault of any kind against women and men is one of the worst types of abuse that human beings can inflict on each other. It is imperative to know that this unwanted, abusive action can cause the victim to experience a deep level of long-term psychological trauma. This trauma is overwhelmingly numbing and painful as it is not warranted and is just a product of someone else's dark desires.

My rape experience conjured a state of confusion, shame, subordination, and fear. These unhealthy emotions stemming from unwanted sexual acts can adversely affect an individual's personality. The impact of this behavioral crisis can not only be devastating but can linger in the subconscious mind for a lifetime. These fearful emotions are so rooted and dominant in the subconscious mind that they can dictate and affect every decision in the individual's life.

Among these decisions lies the raising of children, which can be seriously impacted by an assault victim's emotional triggers. Majority of the time, persons who suffer from Rape Trauma Syndrome will raise their children from a place of fear. This could stem from their desperate need to protect their children from what they had experienced in life.

Over the years, the stigma encircling sexual assault and the act itself has silenced so many people into paralyzing fear, so much that some will never speak to anyone about it due to the embarrassment they are taught to embody on the subject. This state of mind usually goes a long way in breaking the victim's self-esteem, and instead of talking about it, they become set on carrying the secret with them to their graves. Sometimes, nevertheless, some courageous people will shake things up by telling their stories of sexual abuse regardless of the consequences and societal stigma.

I appreciate all the brave people who risked their lives and careers to tell the truth about the rape and unwanted sexual advancement they went through. I guess it got to the point where the courageous souls didn't care about the scrutiny of the public after sharing their stories to the world. They only wanted to do the right thing and free themselves from the shame-prison they feel helplessly bound to. They got sick and tired of what has been the norm for sexual offenders for too long. The #MeToo movement's establishment helped so many survivors realize that they were not alone.

There are certainly some strange moments in time when a victim's truth will catalyze a series of positive campaigns for victims everywhere. One such movement occurred on May 25, 2020, after George Floyd's murder by a police officer in front of the world. His murder caused a significant uproar, one that engulfs the fact that he died at the hands of the very people who were paid to serve and protect him. This action resulted in global demonstrations and a call for police reform.

It also reinforced the Black Lives Matter struggle for equality and fairness for everyone. Finally, when the televisions and smartphones premiered the murder worldwide, it was undeniable to all who saw the picture that this was wrong of former officer Derek Chauvin to kneel on George Floyd's neck over nine minutes as he took his last breath. It took George Floyd's death for the world to understand what Black Lives Matter meant when they speak about inequality, brutality, and unjust treatment by the police.

Similarly, during the 1960s and 1970s, the women's rights movement was born. Like the Black Lives Matter movement, persons, women, in particular, wanted equal rights, opportunities, freedom, the right to choose, pay equity, and much more. The woman's right to choose, an aspect of this movement, is still a struggle for women today.

The movement that helped me and so many others escape our prison of shame was the #MeToo movement. That said, it is unfortunate to learn that a small percentage of women have chosen to use such a significant action for purposes that are not relevant to its intended goal.

However, for the most part, the #MeToo movement gave many people a platform to break free from the shame of sexual assault by telling their stories without feeling blamed or judged. One of the things that were so successful in the #MeToo movement was that the public ended up seeing the abuser in a negative light. For many years, it was the victims who sat on that disgraceful chair.

Finally, the table turned, shattering to pieces and revealing the truth about who should really hide in shame. The table was demolished and stomped on by frustrated yet courageous women who decided it was time to flip the script. One day, one woman finally said enough was enough, and the #MeToo movement was born.

And this 'shame the victim behavior', which was written many years ago by God-knows-who, was finally on its way out. This old biased script of shaming the victim of rape was in place for far too long, gnawing at the victim's subconsciousness, setting them down in a dark corner of guilt and shame. The perpetrators who wrote the 'shame the victim' script intended to embarrass the survivor who suffered a sexual violation into silence. As long as the survivor felt ashamed, it was unlikely that she would speak about the rape to anyone.

Since the #MeToo movement started, the attackers had to jostle around as they tried to hide their shame. It is as if, quite suddenly, the abuser's legs got broken by their own shame, leaving them desperately trying to figure out if they can find at least one leg left to stand upon.

Finally, rather than survivors walking with their heads down in shame, hoping against the odds that no one will ever know they are the victims of sexual assault, they could now become a part of the #MeToo movement for a change.

Karma, in the form of the victim's resilience, visited and right the wrong, and now it is the abusers who are ashamed. Naturally, the abusers turn to the hope that nobody will discover their lousy behavior and in many instances, they walk tall and courageous. This is because as long as the victims are kept quiet by their trauma and shame, the perpetrators are assured protection and can continue to repeat the same evil behavior.

Ever since we flipped the shame script from the survivors to the attackers, they are now the ones hoping against hope that no one will discover the sins of their sexual misconduct against others. All the years of emotional abuse has now set its course in another direction. The shoe is now on the other foot where it belongs, and they are the ones who feel ashamed, and for a good reason as they deserve it.

There are still some guilty abusers hiding in the shadows, protected for several reasons. One of these reasons could be the survivor's continued fear of reporting them—with their main reasons for apprehension stemming from the work environment. Women are most likely to suffer economically, and they are more likely to feel trapped and continue to work in an unsafe environment.

Suppose you are an employee who reads this and you are experiencing some sexual misconduct at work, this #MeToo atmosphere can afford you the platform to voice your concerns about the sexual misconduct you are experiencing. If you are enduring continuous sexual assault in the workplace from another employee, please contact your supervisor immediately. If you are unaware, sexual harassment in the workplace is a violation of the law. I know that the reality surrounding the fear of job loss is genuine and could prevent the worker from revealing that the boss, for example, misbehaves. However, it is paramount that the attacker is held accountable for their actions.

The fear of losing a job is especially true if the worker is the only breadwinner in the household. If that is the case, the worker might think the safest thing to do is keep quiet in order to avoid ruffling any feathers. This is especially true if the victim is the head of a single-parent family household. I can understand that it would put a single parent in a very delicate situation because she has to feed her family when it comes down to it. Nonetheless, her state of mind in that work environment where she feels trapped while being harassed, day in, day out is quite stressful and far outweighs any job.

It is exceedingly stressful for anyone who finds themselves in that position on the job as their mental health is being compromised. If you are an employee and are experiencing unwanted sexual misconduct in the workplace, no matter how daunting you feel the situation may be, you should immediately report it to the management. It is necessary to stop this behavior as soon as it starts. I was a single mother at one point in my life, so I can understand the fear of being unable to support your family. Fortunately for me, I have never been the victim of an inappropriate sexual offence on the job. Luckily, I have been self-employed for almost my entire professional life.

In any case, if that's your story, if you can relate to the aforementioned situation, please tell somebody. Do it for your mental well-being; tell anyone, from a co-worker to the owner of the company. If your boss is also the owner, the last thing he/she wants is for the company to be sued for sexual harassment. They have a legal obligation to ensure your safety.

In reality, if the boss is involved in a sexual harassment situation and you report them, they might try to make your professional life challenging. That is why, in the meantime, you should be looking for new employment immediately while taking the necessary steps to build up a strong case against the company. Document everything, from the actual event you experienced to the date and time it occurred, who witnessed the incident, if applicable, and exactly where you were at the time of the incident. Lastly, speak to the Human Rights Commission.

We are our brother's keeper, and if you leave without taking any action against this company/individual, you are doing great harm to the other employees he/she is hiring. They are in danger of being subjected to the same abusive behavior. In the meantime, you need to get out of that harsh work environment as fast as you can. Ultimately, if you decide to go ahead with your story and are the only breadwinner in your family, your first step is to find a new job.

Consequently, if you are a victim of any workplace violence, I advise you not to surrender your power forever by remaining silent. I know that it is difficult to find the courage to denounce such violence; take all the time you need to become courageous and powerful. You may not be in a position to talk about the sexual misconduct you are experiencing at the moment, but as soon as you feel safe enough to do so, you should free yourself from that abusive behavior.

When that happens, I can promise you that you will be much better off physically, emotionally, and psychologically. Once you dare talk about any sexual harassment you are experiencing, you will feel so free and powerful, and the feeling of freedom and power is your authentic self. You will finally be able to live your life fearlessly once you unveil your soul to the world. You should ensure that your self-unloading is for you, don't do it for anyone else. If you do, the benefits and accomplishments won't feel liberating.

Talk about your unwanted sexual advancement on your terms; allow your spirit to be your guide. The truth is that it will undoubtedly create a significant improvement in your well-being when you no longer have a deep-seated secret weighing you down. I experienced that level of comfort and peace when I expounded on what had happened to me.

The #MeToo movement was the starting point of a campaign that disgraced many sex offenders. One of the great things about the fall of many sexual abusers is that they fell from top to bottom harshly. Some of them fell head first, feet in the air while for some, there was no common ground for a rebound, there was no cushion to soften the blow. And rightly so, they deserved what they got.

Some people will call it karma because they believe that whatever you put into the universe will return to you. This principle honors the idea that if you are good to other people, then you will be rewarded with good things happening in your life. And if you're evil to others, then the same will apply to your life. Do to others what you would like them to do to you; it is not that difficult to respect one another.

There is only one emotion that we should all try to find within ourselves, and that emotion will make a massive difference in the way we treat others in the world. This single emotion is called LOVE. If you have to learn to love, one way to practice is to look at everybody as an extension of your family members because they are. The cultural shift around unwanted sexual assault allows the abusers to be the ones who are ashamed of their actions - finally. That is great for a change and I believe we are on the right path. Unfortunately, shame is not the only emotion that the survivors suffer after the sexual assault.

The initial rape is only one part of the suffering experienced by survivors of sexual assault, so it is great to know that perpetrators are finally receiving some punishment for their actions. Sexual offenders eventually got what they deserved for the selfish use of their masculine power to exploit and take advantage of women. That selfish behavior has changed the course of so many lives forever. They have no idea or concern about the long-term impact of the trauma on the individuals they target.

The abusers who suffer from shame have also had financial hardship because of job loss due to their sexual harassment or rape charges. Depending on their occupations, some of them have lost hundreds of thousands of dollars of income. Furthermore, when it becomes known that they are sexual abusers, it can become increasingly difficult for them to find another job.

The actions of these courageous women, who were not afraid to blow the whistle on some prominent men, opened the door for more victims to share their stories. The first whistle-blowers helped so many women and men realize that it was okay to talk publicly about the unwanted sexual advances they suffered. These daring people who have not been afraid to speak publicly about their ordeal can rest assured that they have genuinely helped the rest of the world, including me.

We realize that if those high-profile sexual abusers can fall from grace, it must mean that their "Time's-Up," as Oprah Winfrey had said in her speech. Time's up seemed befitting in this present climate. I didn't want to miss this opportunity of joining the #MeToo brand of greats, which had inspired me to make a decision and give you my story in writing. I took the opportunity to finally speak about how I became trapped in the shame and guilt that enveloped my life after a gang rape as a child.

The #MeToo Freed Me from My Shame

Usually, when most siblings get together and socialize, they would reminisce about the many childhood memories they shared. Similarly, we recalled and shared past memories when we got together, and we usually enjoyed talking about the fun times we had growing up. But my sister and I had a gloomy cloud hanging over us during these discussions, a big secret that we had never shared with our fellow brothers and sisters. Most of the time, we engage in colorful conversations that encompass the good moments, not the bad ones.

Growing up with my siblings, I never talked about the worst childhood memory that one of my sisters and I suffered together. I've never discussed this secret with anyone until now. I'm going to speak about it in its entirety in this book, disclosing the burden that stood over me in the dark, forcing me into silence. I never talked about the day my sister and I got violently raped in our home; we got raped on beds that we shared with our other siblings. No one in our family knew that one of my sisters and I bore the burden of a terrible secret all our lives. It's a secret I carried around with me from the day it happened. Now, I am finally ready to share it here.

Nobody knew that we were victims of gang rape, which happened to us when we were children. And it's bad enough that it happened to us, but it was done to us by two people from our neighborhood. Like many victims of sexual assault, I experienced the initial emotion of being in shock that it happened, and shortly after that, I experienced shame and sadness.

Girls who are survivors of gang rape are considered bad girls. The shame of being raped, the confusion, and the question of "what did we do wrong?" are some of the thoughts and emotions that many of us have experienced. Also, one of the fears which weighed extremely heavily on me was the fear of the secret being revealed.

The worst part of having been raped was that we suffered in silence. After our traumatic rape experience, the impact, and embarrassment of our ordeal led us to remain silent. We never talked about what went on that day, not even to each other. The dysfunctionality of how that sounds baffles me. However, we pretended as if the rape had never happened by never being vocal about it. At Least this way, we could disassociate from our trauma for some time.

We looked as normal as all our other friends on the outside, but make no mistake that our lives changed that day. We were no longer two innocent young girls; the shame of being raped had destroyed my self-esteem. The rape changed my personality; I felt I wasn't important anymore and like I no longer mattered. While the psychological disturbances were happening in my head, I remained silent on the rape action. It was as if talking about it was proof it had happened. I felt that if I stayed quiet, then I didn't have to believe it. But the conflict I was wrestling with was the rape trauma. I couldn't get rid of the tape playing back the movie of what happened over and over in my head.

While I continued to live a somewhat "normal" life, I suffered from fear and anxiety. One of the main reasons I kept silent about this was the shame directed at rape victims. Shame on the way we believe we would be seen and judged by our peers. We were afraid that if we were to disclose what the two rapists did to us, we would be looked down on and perceived as less than who we were.

Even though we were young girls when the rape occurred, for one reason or another, we already knew of the secret and shame associated with rape survivors. Nobody took us aside and taught us the reality of what was required of us if we ever experienced rape. It was as if we inherently knew we had to keep it a secret. You would think that we were born knowing the fake story that the shame of rape belongs to the rape victim. It was not only the shame of the rape that haunted me, but I felt disrespected and violated even before the rape ended. I'm not quite sure how to explain it, but I'm going to try to explain it as best I can.

It wasn't just the terrible physical pain of the rape itself that we suffered that day, but it was pretty awkward to watch as each of us was raped. You have to realize that we were kids, and the last thing a young girl wanted was for anyone to see her nakedness. You can imagine what we felt when not only were we raped by one rapist that day but two, who looked at our nudity. I had no control over my own body. I was so embarrassed at that moment; I just wanted to die.

The shame alone of this experience was as if I died instantly and sank into the ground. It wasn't a pleasant feeling; it felt like I was going through an out-of-body experience and looking at the occurrence. All I can say is that it was a terrible thing for a child to go through, and I don't wish this to happen to anyone.

Unfortunately, one shameful stigma that will continue to silence a person who experiences rape is the fear of being considered a damaged commodity. This stigma will sadly keep survivors of rape silent for a very long time. One of our problems was that we were afraid of how others would perceive us if they knew about the secret. So, we both chose to remain silent without even having a conversation about it with each other.

We both made this decision without having any collaboration between us. It was as if we were on a code, already aware of the secret drill.

Another strange thing about the surreal situation was that both rapists didn't even need to threaten us not to say anything to anyone. They weren't afraid to get caught. They didn't have to tell us to keep quiet, or they would harm our family, as you see in the movies. We knew what we needed to do, to protect our reputation no matter what.

They didn't have to tell us anything; they were confident we would keep it a secret. Both rapists knew that we would not dare talk to anyone about what they did to us, or we would be disgraced. We knew our peers would vilify us if anyone found out about the secret. Although we were children, we were female first, and in my mind, this is what happens to women.

The silent code among girls and women is that we should keep sexual misconduct quiet for fear of being labeled bad girls by men and women. This code automatically protects the rapist; it is like a silent code, and every girl knows how to play within this code of silence. This unwritten rule is that if you become a victim of any sexual violation in your life, you should not talk to anybody about it; otherwise, you would be vilified. These same little girls become adult women who continue to live under the same code and continue to keep the secret of sexual assault to themselves. My sister and I have proven to be the epitome of this "code silence".

It would seem that we are born knowing that we will have to face sexual assault at some point in our lives as females. And when sexual assault happens to us, we should keep quiet or be punished. It was a constant reminder that this is a man's world, and women were second-class citizens. In my opinion, rape is the most degrading act that can happen to anyone, and the shame of it results in the victim remaining silent, which keeps the perpetrator safe. Since the #MeToo movement began, however, our cries are finally being heard. It's a blessing for everyone.

Sometimes a few women would go to the police and go to court. However, when that happens, the women are challenged in the courtroom to prove what happened to them. They would need to recall every detail of the incident to prove their case.

They need to remember everything from the color of the dress they wore that day to whether their hair was in a bun or not. In the event that the accuser denies that the rape occurred, then the victim has to prove her court case, which can be pretty challenging for her. Over the years, it's become a deterrent for other women, especially if the victim couldn't prove her case due to "his word against hers".

Lenore Lukasik-Foss, who heads the Ontario Coalition of Rape Crisis Centers, said, "Because of the kinds of questioning that the defense uses, some survivors say it's re-traumatizing for them." She said, "Victims are afraid to report rape because of the fear of going to court only to be blamed and shamed."

According to Statistics Canada, there are four hundred and sixty thousand sexual offenses each year. And for every one thousand incidents, only thirty-three are reported, twelve result in charges, six go to trial, and three lead to a conviction. These findings are not very encouraging for women to report rape.

These are some of the reasons why sex offenders feel very confident that they can get away with their crimes.

When it comes to offenders, if the woman chooses to go to court, they will deny that the rape happened. And she'll feel as if she's on trial to prove her case. For these reasons, the very idea of going to court will silence most rape survivors.

The two rapists who raped my sister and me didn't have to tell us not to tell anybody. We automatically knew that we had to keep quiet for our sake. We knew that it should stay between the four of us. I often wondered how we knew that and when exactly did that information get downloaded and integrated into our young minds.

Undoubtedly, the silent code works very well for the rapist; it's become some security blanket for them. It provided an opportunity for them to use the victim's silence as a safety net, and this security makes it possible for them to move on to the next target.

After we got raped, it was a somber and depressing period for me. The worst part of it was that we couldn't support each other. We were young and shy and didn't know how to start a conversation about the gang rape we experienced. And because we were embarrassed to talk about it, we couldn't support each other morally, so we suffered alone.

We are now adults, and I still don't know exactly how this affected my sister emotionally because she never told me about her suffering. For me, the only thing I can say is that after what I saw and endured physically and emotionally, I still don't know how we even functioned in society without any form of psychological counseling.

After the traumatic rape, I had trouble trusting people, especially men. This impacted my self-worth for a very long time. However, I eventually learned to live with my situation by suppressing those despicable memories. When I became a young adult, I left Jamaica and migrated to live in Canada. I was happy about the move for many reasons, but one reason was that nobody in Canada knew about my embarrassing childhood story. In this case, I have a new beginning to focus all my attention on the return of my self-confidence, personal value, and self-esteem.

The only two people other than the two rapists that knew what happened to us were my sister and me. And both rapists were not residents of Canada. It was a chance for me to learn to hold my head up high and stand tall again. I'm not going to say it was easy because it took me quite a while to gain my confidence back. By taking one step at a time, over the years, I eventually regained my self-worth.

The #MeToo movement gave me the courage I needed to tell my story and free myself from my childhood imprisonment. I always wanted to tell my children this part of my childhood, but I did not dare to do it because of the shame. Although I am lucky to have three of the most loving and understanding children in the world, I still could not tell them the secret of my childhood rape which haunted me for decades.

I didn't know how to tell my kids something so painful, and another thing is that I didn't want to go back to that terrible day, as I would have to relive the experience to write about it. I just wasn't ready emotionally. How can I begin a conversation like this? I had no idea where to start this difficult conversation with them. But, help was on the way; it was called #MeToo.

I felt free and empowered; it was time to talk about my entire childhood life to my children. Before the movement, when I spoke to them about my childhood memories, I used to leave out the rape part of my story. I left it blank because I couldn't verbalize something so painful to them. The memory stayed in my subconscious mind and I used it to measure the various decisions I had to make in my life. Especially decisions that had to do with my children.

Subsequently, moving forward, that day shaped how I lived my life. It is prominent in many aspects of my decision-making. I raised my children with the paranoia of constantly protecting them from the evil I experienced. I didn't want anybody to hurt them the way I was hurt. My sister and I didn't have anyone to save us that day, so I made sure my kids were always protected.

I will say that it may have seemed that I was a bit too protective of them on certain occasions. Well, I must admit, I was overprotective of my children. But I would rather be considered an overprotective mother and keep them safe than not be there if something were to happen and they needed my help.

Sadly, the anxiety I suffered from my childhood sexual assault has caused me to parent my children from a place of fear. I was an overly sensitive mom, especially when it came to my children's welfare and safety. I was always afraid that somebody might rape them, and so, I had to protect them. My children are all grown up now, and I still get concerned about their safety, even to this day.

I always had to make sure that my kids were safe from sex predators. As a result, I did everything I could to protect them. First, I continuously resided with them; I knew I could never abandon my responsibility to raise them. My mother didn't raise us, and I remembered being angry because my mother wasn't there to protect me and my sister from the horrible ordeal we went through that day.

Although I always knew I wanted to talk about the terrible day I got raped in our house, I was afraid of how it would be perceived. So, when the familiar dialogue began, in Hollywood, and all the movie stars went out and told their stories, I knew if I didn't do it at the time, the wave would pass, and my story would remain on the shelf where it would still be sitting and waiting to be told. So I decided to tell my children by writing it down for them. I wanted them to know how it affected me in my adult life and how it ultimately affected their lives.

I Cried for Her, and Then I Cried for Me

I started by crying for my sister, and I had no idea that my tears would soon be shed for myself. I was right there, I witnessed everything that was happening, yet I could not help her. I was so young and naive that I didn't even know I was about to go through the same fate as her, next in line to deal with what she'd just gone through. And the trauma wasn't over for her either, because the second rapist still needed his turn with her.

When I was raising my children, I got a chance to use their age to compare to when I got raped at that age. I came to the realization that I was a kid when it happened. We didn't even understand that some ruthless people exist in the world who will hurt children just because they can. We were only children when the two inhumane rapists changed the course of our lives forever.

The rape happened when we were living in Jamaica, in the parish of Clarendon. Our district consisted of three different sections. One of our rapists lived in our section, the other in another section adjoining ours. We lived in the countryside on the island. A twenty-minute walk was not a big deal to us, unlike the city people, who would make a fuss if they had to walk for ten minutes; they would think it too far to walk. In essence, the two rapists were within walking distance of our house; we could say that one of them lived just around the corner. In any event, we were all from the same community in Clarendon, with one of them residing in a different section.

We heard that our district got a portion of its name by having a lot of corn grass back then. I don't want to identify the community in Clarendon, Jamaica, where we lived at the time. This is due to the fact that I still have relatives there and I do not want any problems for them. For this reason, in addition, I won't identify the two rapists; I can say that our district had an animal's nickname that is added to one section's known name.

We heard one section of our community got its nickname because several donkeys were there from our ancestors' time. Another name for donkey as used by the district's inhabitants was Jack-horse (Jackass in Jamaican creole). Therefore, the community informally alluded to Jackass when saying the official name of one section.

Nowhere has it been written that Jackass is a part of the district's name but rather a passive reference to one section. For clarity, residents have used it to differentiate between the two sides of the same neighborhood. It was helpful for the residents because now they could further differentiate between both sides of the community instead of referring to them as having the same name. The first rapist lived on the district's side where Jackass got associated with; we also lived on that side. The second rapist lived on the other side of the community. He, therefore, lived right around the corner from where we were living. With that being said, I will not mention any more information about the district's name.

Coming from a small community like ours, most people knew one another. Sometimes you may not be aware of the names of some of the people you've seen, but you will most likely recognize that you have seen their faces before. Our property had no immediate neighbors on both sides at the time; the neighboring properties had only fruit trees and bushes. So our house was somewhat isolated in regards to our neighbors. The property behind ours was that of our cousin, with the front of their house facing another street. The end of their land was attached to the end of ours.

In any case, a neighbor's house was directly in front of our home. But we were so unfortunate that no one was there on the day the horrible incident happened. It was regrettable that our mom no longer lived with us at the family home the day the incident occurred, or she would be able to protect her children. The relationship between her and our father was over, and he raised us all on his own. It was an abusive relationship, so she moved out of the house many years before our violent rape.

Our single father, who had raised us, was at work when it happened. Like most single working parents, he had to work to support his family. So, all of this happened when my single father was at work, and my younger siblings were in school. The incident that occurred that day changed my life forever.

I will give an overview of how the event began. One of my older sisters and I were the only people at home that day. I believe I was between twelve and fourteen years old, and my sister was two years older than I was. I was not at school for a brief time because I had just returned to live with my father after living with my mother for a few years. My mother had moved to another district further away, and that district was where I went to school before returning to live with my father.

After returning home to live with my father and my siblings, I told him I didn't want to go back to my neighborhood school. The original school I attended while living with my mother was too far away for me to travel back and forth every day. So I was at home awaiting the start of my new school in September of that year.

One of my older sisters, whom my younger siblings and I loved and adored, had just come back to live in our neighborhood after living in Saint Catherine with our aunt and uncle. Saint Catherine is among the fourteen parishes of Jamaica but we were born and raised in Clarendon.

It was our mother who decided to send my sister to live with our aunt and uncle. This aunt was the wife of our uncle, who was our mother's brother. My sister moved in with them shortly after the breakup of our mom and dad's relationship. My father didn't like that decision, but it was initiated and acted upon without his consent.

My uncle, who was going to Canada to work, wanted my sister to assist his wife in caring for their children while he was away. Because my sister was older, they needed her to help them with their younger children. At that time, the older children were more willing to help out than the younger children. It's not so much like that nowadays.

I should take the time to tell you that our father would never agree to send my sister to live with our uncle. He said that he would never allow any of his children to be gifted to anybody. Whether it is a family member or not, he would generally say that his children were not puppies to give to anyone.

The turn of events began when our aunt decided to migrate to Canada to reunite with her husband. It was then that my sister and cousins, the children of my aunt and uncle, were returned to our district to live with my aunt's mother. And my sister kept living with my aunt's mom and continued to help with my young cousins.

All I can say is that it was a different time; my sister was herself a child who still needed a parental guardian. My uncle's mother-in-law looked after her well-being while she lived with them nevertheless. Somebody had to because she was just a child herself. If she was old enough to look after the children independent of an adult, she certainly could have stayed back in Saint Catherine and raised them without any supervision. I just wanted to point out that she was still a child who needed a parental guardian.

My sister was very cheerful, good-natured, and friendly. She was the one with the social butterfly personality and as a result, she was very popular. They not only knew her through facial recognition, they knew her by name.

Our mother named my sister in honor of her mother, our grandma, whom none of us had the good fortune to meet because, unfortunately, she passed away before we were born. When you compare her personality to mine, I was more reserved and shy, and I didn't warm up to people as quickly as she did. The extrovert and friendly character of my sister made it easier for her to make friends. Her personality had made her many friends, but the downside is that she trusted everyone who had befriended her.

I was more cautious with people than my sister; maybe I couldn't put it into words, but deep inside, I knew that the world is not only filled with good people. Sadly, some bad people are mixed in with the good ones. For those reasons, I didn't trust people as quickly as she did. And, as I was somewhat shy, I didn't talk to everyone, and I didn't befriend everyone as opposed to my sister. I didn't have as many friends as she did due to my reserved personality, but I didn't mind. I liked it better when I had a few trusted friends to connect with on a deeper level compared to having many casual friends. My few good friends were enough for me.

However, I must admit that I sometimes benefited from the fact that everyone knew my sister. It worked for me especially if somebody was trying to identify who I was. I would mention her name and tell them that she was my sister, and they would place me immediately. For that reason, having an outgoing sister was pretty cool.

The Day My Life Changed Paths

Let me elaborate on what happened to my sister and me on the infamous day of the rape. Living on the island, we can expect to have any of these weathers: sunny, cloudy, or rainy. Sometimes we would even have all three combined, but you will not see snow on the ground as we have here in Canada and many other parts of the world.

Just before the rape occurred, the day unfolded like any other day. A distant, radiant sun emerged from the east, like any other waking hours, warming the island and commencing the day. There was nothing out of the ordinary as the day progressed. My sister came to visit as usual; the only difference that day compared to other times when she came to visit was that I was the only one at home. All my other siblings were in school, so it turned out that she came to see me that day. We talked and laughed together, and we were having a lovely time just before the two devils showed up.

We were hanging out in the front yard as we had done on numerous occasions with our siblings and sometimes with our friends. It was typical for families to sit around in the front yard and socialize with their friends and family when growing up. There was nothing wrong with having two girls sitting outside their home in Jamaica. For the most part, on the island, everybody takes care of one another.

My sister lived within walking distance of our family house, so it was neither unusual nor difficult for her to visit us as often as she wanted. As a result, she came to see us several times a week, and this visit was one of her many visits.

The first rapist was a well-known cyclist in our community and he was kind of a local celebrity in our area. He was known as an excellent cyclist who won several bicycle races. He was also known for his cooking; this is because, admittedly, he was a great cook.

So, not only was he famous in our community, and everybody knew him by name, he was also known and admired by many people in our surrounding communities. Everyone knew him and admired him for his sportsmanship and charisma. He had a powerful voice when speaking, and some might even say that he had a vulgar personality.

He was an outstanding cyclist, the one to watch out for in all the local cycling races. He was always the favorite; of course, he was a very competitive and determined cyclist. We could rely on him to win races for our community. And our district was very proud of him for competing for us.

Let's get back to the series of events that led to the rape. It was not strange for "rapist-one" to ride past our house on his bicycle several times per day. But on that day, as he was going by, he spotted my sister, which prompted him to stop. When I say our home, I'm talking about the home I lived in with my single father and four other siblings. I should mention that the first rapist house was on the same street as ours. It was within walking distance.

As I said earlier, the sister I was hanging out with that day did not live with us at that time. She still lived with our aunt's mother in a neighboring district a little further away from our family home but within walking distance. The route going past our house was his regular route, but he could use another road depending on his destination. It was his shortest route if he wanted to go to the other side of our district. He could have taken a few other streets, but the road going past our home was the shortest one.

When he spotted my friendly and outgoing sister, he called out to her and then immediately turned his bicycle around. He stood up from his bicycle seat as he pedaled his way towards our gate. My sister walked towards the gate to speak to him, which she had done several other times before that day. Everyone talked to my sister, including him. He would stop and talk to her several times before that day, so it was not odd for them to talk.

He was a member of our community, he was no stranger, and he was someone we knew all our lives. As mentioned, the house he and his family lived in was on the same street as ours. He lived a few homes away from us, so he was no stranger to us. He was our local celebrity.

Everything happened so quickly on that horrible day. Honestly, I was so frightened that I can't perfectly remember how it all happened in sequence. I can only say that the first rapist was joined quickly by a second rapist who was also a community member. The second rapist, like the first rapist, was from our district and was not a stranger to us, and he knew who we were. He lived a bit further away than the first rapist, but he still lived within walking distance. He lived in another section of our neighborhood, and listen to this: his father was friends with our father.

As the first rapist had a conversation with my sister, I don't remember paying much attention to them as they stood and spoke to each other. It wasn't until my sister started screaming for him to let her go that I looked in their direction. It was then that I noticed that she was trying to break free from his grip. I saw that he had his claws holding her by the hand as he tried to drag her towards our house.

My sister was screaming and trying to get out of his clutch. I looked in their direction and yelled for him to let her go. I approached him and attempted to stop him. He didn't want to listen to me; he was determined to get her into our house. He was in front of her as he dragged her very hard, pulling her towards the house.

While the first rapist pulled my sister towards our house, I pulled her backward; I tried to pull her away from our home. I suppose I became a bit of an annoyance to him by pulling her back. I desperately wanted to help my sister escape from him, but I failed because I wasn't strong enough.

As we cried and begged him to stop, he would not listen to us. Our tears never mattered to him; they were hopeless tears. He desperately wanted to do whatever it took to get my sister into the house, and I desperately tried everything I could to prevent him from succeeding.

I was not about to give up on my sister; I went after him like a dog fighting for a bone. I was fierce, I hit and punched him, and he acted as if he had no feelings whatsoever, as if my punches meant nothing to him. He soon got help when the second rapist showed up and joined forces with him instead of helping us. As I struggled to free my sister from his grip, it was then that the second rapist arrived on his bicycle, and I soon realized that he had not come to help us.

He quickly jumped off his bicycle and grabbed me by my arm right away; he held my arm so tight as if he wanted to let me know that he would break it if that's what it took for me to cooperate with them. I realized that the more I got mad and tried to get away from him, the tighter his grip became on my arm.

The intensity of his restraint caused me to calm a little and stop trying to get away. At that point, the one thing I could do was watch with horror as our lives changed in an instant. My sister and I had just hung out and chatted like everyone else in our neighborhood. We didn't do anything wrong, and within minutes, we were under siege by these two giant rapists with no conscience.

We were no match for them, so of course, we lost the battle. I felt disabled and powerless, and the fear of what was happening was unbearable. It seemed that the only thing my sister and I could do at this point was to weep and begged them to stop. But all our begging and crying went on deaf ears. There was no point in trying anymore, we were at their mercy, and our screams were hopeless. They were not about to let us go because the stakes were too high. The prize was the opportunity to rape two kids instead of one.

Once they were inside our house, they acted as if they were responsible for our lives. They were our owners, so they could do whatever they wanted to do to us. It was as if we were the slaves in which they had bought to torture. I realized at this point that begging didn't work, and trying to escape using our physical strength was impossible. All I could think about at the time was that the second rapist restrained me, and I was unable to help my desperate and screaming sister. And she was incapable of helping me; in essence, we were unable to help each other.

The two rapists were adults, they were physically very strong rapists and they were determined to do whatever they wanted with us. We were incapable of overpowering both of them; it wasn't going to happen. At that point, we would have needed a miracle to assist us. The only thing I could think about was: "why couldn't this be one of those days when my father came home early from work?" For some reason, on that day, everything worked out to the two rapists' advantage. We were alone at home, there was no one to defend us, and our siblings were not due home for lunch until a few hours later.

While I was being held captive by the second rapist, my thoughts were that he would let me go after his rapist friend finished raping my sister. For the whole time, I just thought he was doing his friend a favor by holding me back. I thought he wanted his friend to rape my sister without being interrupted by me hitting him. I could not even fathom the level of suffering that was in store for us both. In my child's mind at the time, I thought that the second rapist had detained me because he thought I was causing too many problems by hitting his friend to separate my sister from him.

Under no circumstance could I anticipate what was about to happen next. I had no idea that the day that began so well would have unfolded in both of us getting gang-raped in our home. Both rapists came from our neighborhood, my dad was friends with the dad of the second rapist, how could I have known that he would restrain me until his friend finished raping my crying sister? I had no idea it would be my turn to be tormented afterward. The rapist who initiated the rape was a local cyclist. He had won several cycling races for our neighborhood before the rape. He, of course, continued to cycle and competed with other bikers after the rape.

Naturally, he continued his whole life as if he had done nothing wrong, and he still won several more races. The rape had never affected any sexual offenders emotionally, psychologically, or physically. They usually get to live out their dreams without any sexual trauma whatsoever—this daring behavior by sex offenders is unacceptable and unfair to the rape survivors. Sexual abusers can ruin the lives of as many people as they want and then they can go about their business and live their lives to their full potential. Rapists can do as they please without having to endure the trauma and shame of being raped. They can enjoy every day of their lives without any mental disruption, trauma, or the overall devastation of rape.

On the other hand, rape causes emotional and psychological trauma for the survivors for the rest of their life. For the most part, the lives of survivors have changed forever. Rape survivors typically suffer from the enduring shame of being raped.

Often, the bicycle race would be on the street, and when that happened, the people in our district who were into sports would gather along both sides of the road. They would line the street so they could catch a glimpse of the first rapist and cheered him on as he rode past our roadside gathering.

As I looked back, while trying to recall the personality of both rapists, I can't imagine the kind of person you would have to be in order to inflict these types of cruel acts on one another. How can two adults have the same sort of non-compassionate heart? They could both team up and viciously rape two young girls without any feeling of guilt or kindness.

Both rapists got away with what they did to us without any consequence for the bad behavior, while for us, that day changed our lives forever. They never needed to think about it, not even as a flashback in the back of their minds.

For them, it was just water under the bridge. But for me, the rape memory became a part of my story.

Sexual offenders can live their life and forget the rape in which they were involved. But survivors like my sister and I were deprived of living our lives without the experience of rape as a part of our journey. I often wondered what my life would have been like emotionally if I didn't have to suffer through rape. I can only imagine what a life without the rape experience is like, but I will never know for sure.

As well, do you realize that survivors of rape are dysfunctional sometimes? In some cases, a rape survivor can continue to remain friends with a rapist for several months or even years after the rape. This is particularly true if they got raped by somebody they knew. I can only say you never know what the shame after getting raped will make you do. An example of this would be after my traumatic rape experience with this cyclist rapist, I continued to cheer for and encouraged him to win races for our community. This dysfunctional action also helped cover up the rape, but unfortunately, it facilitated and protected the rapists.

Questions for the Rapists

I have several questions for both rapists to which I know I might never get the answers, but just having the opportunity to write my questions here is enough for me.

Questions for the first rapist:

1. What was happening in both your twisted heads that led you to believe that my sister and I wanted to get rape?
2. What made you so sure raping young girls was a good thing to do?
3. What prompted you two to gang-rape two innocent young girls? My God, we were two scared young girls; who does that?
4. What kind of animals were you two?
5. What sort of distorted mentality, deranged monster does one have to be not to feel empathy for children crying out in pain and knowing full well that you both were responsible for their suffering?

Questions for the second rapist:

1. Why did you hold me back until your rapist friend raped my sister before you gave me to him for him to go ahead and rape me as well?
2. Was the whole thing just a sick orchestrated game for you two?
3. Why did you hold on to me only to give me to the first rapist like I was a present for him?
4. Were you planning on raping me earlier that day while you held me captive?
5. You stood there and held me for what seemed like forever. Even though you saw how horrified I was and how I was shaking with fear, why didn't it disturb you in any way?

It bothers me that you didn't show any consideration for our well-being. I hope you're both aware that the selfish decision you made that day traumatized us and left us with some significant emotional scars for the rest of our lives. Why was it essential for you to force me to watch in horror as your rapist friend raped and tortured my sister? And unfortunately, when I thought it was all over, it was my turn to go through the same fate as she just went through.

To the second rapist who held me hostage, more than your rapist friend, you knew how terrified I was because it was you who prevented me from moving while your friend raped my sister. And after what she had just gone through, you still decided to rape her regardless of her well-being.

My sister had just got raped by your rapist friend and was still hurting very badly from the first rape. What made you so cruel and heartless? You both have daughters and women in the family; you have sisters, and you have a mother. How would you feel if you had to watch a couple of rapists attack your mother and sisters?

I often wonder why you were not empathetic towards two frightened young girls. Did you even realize that we had feelings and that the reason we wept was that you two rapists truly hurt us? Or did you think we were rocks and didn't feel anything? I don't want to ask you if you saw us like animals, because animals do have feelings.

And, if that wasn't enough torture you two have put us through for that day, you were still not satisfied. No, you were going to inflict even more pain when you took turns raping two young girls. It's like you decided that we ought to suffer even more physical and emotional ordeal in your twisted mind. So you two chose to use the gang-rape to seal the disgrace.

The degree of disgrace associated with when someone got gang-raped scared us and left us no other choice but to remain silent. The act of getting gang-rape was awful and very damaging to our good character. Did you both select to use the gang-rape method on us so that you could protect the secret? You both knew that the secret could be locked away forever by using that type of rape on us. Both of you knew there isn't a girl in her right mind who would tell the world that they got gang-raped; if that happens, she would be ridiculed and shamed into hiding.

I believe the purpose of you humiliating us the way you did that caused us to suffer physically and psychologically was to keep your secret safe forever. Yes, it made you feel a lot safer knowing the impact of the gang-raped; you knew that it would be much more demeaning to us girls. Thus, you used this strategy to assure both your safety. You used the shame and confusion of the gang-rape action to exploit and manipulate us further.

For these reasons, there is absolutely no way we would want to tell anyone that we were raped, let alone gang-raped. Your plan worked; for many years, your secret was safe for a very long time. Have you noticed that I said your secret? I understand now that it was never our secret in the first place. Rape secrets, whose secrets are they? Until now, I carried your secret around with me because I wasn't brave enough to return it to both of you. But I finally got the bravery when some courageous men and women said, "Enough is Enough" and "Time's Up."

After you handed me over to your rapist friend so I could get raped by him, I was given back to you when he was through with me, and this time it wasn't for you to stand there and restrain me. No, this was so I could be tortured and raped by you as well. What are your thoughts on all that happened that day? Did you feel as if it added to your masculinity? Did you rape us to prove your manhood to the world? If this was the plan, I'm here to tell you that you're not a man, and neither is your rapist friend.

A true man doesn't have to rape anybody to prove his manhood; you are both losers who only had the strength to terrorize young girls. You both targeted children because they aren't physically strong enough to defend themselves against the strong adult-male rapist monsters. That only makes us see both of you for precisely what you are: two hoodlum pussies.

The anguish we both experienced is programmed in our subconscious minds forever and it immediately changed how I see myself existing in the world. I couldn't figure out why we had to suffer at both your hands for not having a mother at home. I felt that rape was a form of punishment for something we had no control over, so I blamed my mother for leaving us unprotected for many years.

It seemed like we should feel regret or guilt that we were born females. I am not suggesting that boys and men are not victims of rape, sexual assault, and sexual harassment; I am very aware that some boys and men experience some form of inappropriate sexual advances and rape. I'm just saying that most sexual assault survivors are women, and in our case, we were a couple of girls.

One of the things that stuck with me the most was after the first rapist raped my sister; both rapist monsters traded us like slaves. The first rapist raped me, and the second rapist also raped me. It was like you two were using us to play a very sick game. And when you were both finished with us, you just casually rode off on your bicycles. It was like it was just another day in the life of two of our neighborhood rapists.

How did you feel when you both rode away on your bicycles and expected the two young sisters you had just tortured with rape to cleaned up your mess? You left us there to clean up the mess you both created? And because we desperately needed to cover up the rape, we had to wash all the messed-up sheets that were in pretty bad condition. And on the island a few decades ago, all laundry was done by hand; there were no washing machines like we have today.

Nowadays, washing machines are more prevalent on the island; it has become a necessity. But, even to this day, many people still do their laundry by hand. However, we had no washing machines and we had to wash our clothes by hand. You can imagine what we were going through at the time. We had just got gang-raped, and we had to stand up on our feet and wash our sheets by hand.

Cleaning the linen was done with the intent of hiding the rape and our shame. But now I know that the shame of the rape belonged to both rapists. It was their shame, it had absolutely nothing to do with us. In my confused child's mind, I thought we caused the rape, that it was our fault. It was embarrassing for me, and we didn't want our father and other siblings to know what had happened.

That was the day the big secret was born, and it was buried deep inside my subconscious mind. I spent every day of every month and every year following that day hiding the secret from everyone.

During a typical laundry day, we usually sat down to wash the clothes by hand. But on the day of the rape, we stood on our feet to do the laundry. That was because we were too sore to sit down on our buttocks. We couldn't sit down because we were in such physical pain following the rape.

Did you feel proud of yourselves for your behavior toward us that day? You left it up to the two young girls you had just raped to clean up after you adult males. How cruel is that? It was unimaginable that you were the so-called adults when you both left a couple of children to figure out how to handle the mess you created.

I often wondered why you let me stand there and watch my sister suffer from being raped, her screams ripping through the essence of my being, echoing against my subconscious, how could you not be disturbed? You felt it necessary to watch, while you bound me, her inhumane suffering from the pain of rape. Was that a turn-on for you? It's a very perverted act, and our tears didn't disturb you enough for you to tell your abusive friend to stop hurting us.

You stood there without any compassion for us, trading us back and forth like mere objects for your nasty desires. The two words that I have for you both are "cold" and "heartless". When I look back on that day, I still can't figure out why you both felt the need to hurt us this way. It was challenging for me to upload these bad memories from my subconscious mind to write this book.

Doing this meant that I had to go back to that forbidden place where those memories were all stored so that I could retrieve them. And going back there put me in that same emotional state as the day of the rape. However, I find it necessary because it was therapeutic; it helped me tremendously with my healing because it allowed me to see clearly now.

One surprising thing to me that day was when the second rapist, Thomas, showed up- oops, I shouldn't have mentioned his name – and when he arrived at the scene, he wasn't there to help us. Your behavior was shocking to me; I must admit that I was frightened when I was seized, subdued, and held tightly by this rapist. His dad was a friend of our dad and for this reason, the whole incident was unexpected and confusing. I was highly disappointed when I realized that your only interest when you came by was to help yourself, torturing us instead of saving us. Do you care to explain what prompted you to choose that action?

I had to reflect on how I was restrained and forced to watch my crying sister in horror as she was being torn apart by the first rapist. This reflection helped me to heal and that subtracted most of the pain I encountered. The second rapist also raped her without any hesitation or concern for her health. And then, it was my turn to go through the same agony as her. To retrieve the rape memories, I can assure you it was not an easy task reliving that awful day. But as mentioned above, it was necessary for my mental health and this book's purpose.

How Your Actions Affected My Psyche

Research shows that unwanted sexual behavior, by its very nature, is designed to cause emotional, physical, moral, and psychological trauma to the victim. From the day I was gang-raped as a child, I suffered from Rape Trauma Syndrome. I felt very happy when I realized that my psychological pain was recognized by society and even given a name. I knew I was affected by the traumatic rape experience, but I didn't know what it was called or that it was institutionalized.

I am now an adult, and it is still challenging for me to take my mind back to that terrible day to write this book. Since the rape took place, this is the first time I have removed these feelings of pain from the filing cabinet they have remained in for decades. I had to make the difficult decision to turn back the clock and tell my story.

When I said that my pain was sitting in the filing cabinet, don't get me wrong, it didn't sit on the shelf collecting dust. The pain came to the front line now and then to act as a dictator when I had to make certain decisions, especially about my children. My fear would make those decisions on my behalf. Since writing this book, it's the first time I could elect to pick up the pain from the shelf it had been sitting on for decades. I decided to gather my mental strength, take it off and face it head-on. I have never really examined the situation in its entirety, only exposed to a glimpse of it when it resurfaces in a memory. I always knew that one day I would have to review it totally to coexist with it as part of my experience.

When I said I put aside my hurt feelings, I meant that I never talked to anyone about it. I became very good at disguising my Rape Trauma Syndrome although I've lived my life in the rape space and raised my children from that place. Many of the decisions I made surrounding my children and my family have been out of that space.

You rapists ought to know that your selfish acts changed our lives that day. It would help if you saw the implication of rape on someone's life after the initial rape. My sister and I are an example of what you put us through when both of you gang-raped us in our home. Since then, the trauma of rape has never left my mind. Through science, we know that the way parents raise their children has a significant influence on what they will become. So the trauma of my rape will not stop with my children; it will affect the second, and possibly, third generation. This is called the grandmother effect. My children will raise their children from that same rape trauma place from which they were raised. I call that place of fear, the rape zone.

You left us broken with many unanswered questions and a sense of shame over what happened to us. Reflecting on what transpired that day, I often wondered what we did to indicate to you two that we wanted to be raped by you. I often thought about what I could have done differently to prevent the life-changing evil of rape from happening to us. My sister and I were embarrassed to talk to each other about that horrible rape we went through together. You can imagine we couldn't even speak to each other about it as the sheer embarrassment damaged our communication process. As a result, the two of us suffered alone in silence. It was unfortunate, at the very least, because we should have become a support system for each other.

We lived with this shame and fear our entire lives. In my mind at the time I would think: God forbid anyone should find out about our gang rape, I would be devastated. For a very long time, I blamed different people for the rape. I secretly blamed my sister, I blamed my mother for not living with us, I blamed myself for not being strong enough to fight the rapist who restrained me and forced me to watch my sister's raped.

And do you know what the worst part was? The worst thing was that there was no way we could avoid seeing the two rapists, day in, day out. After all, how could we not see them? We all lived in the same community. I tried to stay in the backyard more often to avoid seeing them. I felt so embarrassed I never wanted them ever to see me again. It took quite a long time for me to come to grips with that level of shame. I would usually hold my head down to the ground, and could not make eye contact with anyone because I was too ashamed.

Now that the culture has changed around sexual assault and sexual harassment, I am more confident that, as a survivor of rape, I can finally tell my story without being disrespected or judged.

In this book, I finally asked some of the questions I've wanted to ask the rapists all these years. I have an opportunity to speak directly to both rapists in this book and I get a chance to tell them how I feel about them as well.

Being able to speak freely about the horrific gang rape has helped me in my healing process. As we advance, I was able to free myself from the clutches of the rape trauma – "literally". You can never imagine how difficult it was for me to see you, two rapists, as you ride your bicycles past our home. Not to mention the fact that those same bikes you two rapists rode daily were parked in our front yard on the day of the vicious rape. We suffered at the hands of you, two heartless rapists.

I can finally look at the incident now in detail. The more I look at it, the more I can see the intense psychological trauma you've caused us to go through. Your cold-hearted action caused you to disrespect the more intimate part of our lives. We were no match for two strong, ruthless male rapists. How on earth were two young girls supposed to overpower you two?

The Shame, Guilt and Blame

I have lived with this terrible shame ever since the day my sister and I were violently raped in our home by two members of our neighborhood. The humiliation of being sexually violated was appalling; it prevented my sister and me from conversing with each other about the terrible ordeal we endured that day.

We were devastated by the embarrassment and guilt of the pain we suffered so much that the shame of rape caused us to pretend it had never happened. We got so good at pretending that we even pretended to each other that it didn't happen. Shame and guilt are two paralyzing emotions that can unfold into an impotent sense of fear. I'm sure many rape survivors can relate to this description.

Rape shame is the most paralyzing shame that can stay with you even into adulthood. If my sister and I were not so embarrassed to discuss the rape we experienced, we could at least give each other the moral support we both needed. Both rapists had deprived us of the opportunity to live a life without having a rape experience like most other girls. Most girls do not have to live with a rape experience as a part of their childhood. However, we never got that opportunity, we have no idea what that felt like because of the two rapists.

That said, I know that I can speak for my sister when I say the mutual embarrassment for each other is part of what kept us from talking to each other about that day. I was embarrassed for both myself and my sister, and I'm sure the feelings were mutual. One of the things that haunted me for years was that I don't know if my sister felt guilty because of what happened to us that day, but I hope she doesn't.

I said that because she was the one who was talking to the first rapist before the rape occurred. She was the one who the first rapist spotted when he quickly made a U-turn and approached our gate. He wouldn't have turned around if it was just me at home because he and I have never had any conversation before as we were not friends. He used to say hello to me sometimes, but that was it. He and I had never had a real conversation with each other. The only reason the first rapist stopped and turned his bicycle around was because he spotted my sister. Usually, he wouldn't stop when he saw me because we didn't have anything to discuss. He was much older than I was, I was more of an introvert, so what exactly would we have in common to discuss?

He and my sister were having a conversation before he decided to rape her. I was not his intended target, I just got caught up in the mess of it by being in the wrong place at the wrong time. How ironic is this statement? I was at home in my front yard, so where is the right place to escape being raped? I got involved because I went to her defense when he was dragging her towards our house. I have no idea, to this day, if my sister felt guilty about what happened to me, as she and I have never discussed the rape.

After the rape, I blamed my mother for not living with us to protect us as mothers are supposed to do. When she lived with us, she was a stay-at-home mother. For most mothers in our district, staying at home was a common trend.

That is why I knew that she would be at home taking care of her children like all the other mothers in our district did in those days. In that case, she would have been home that day to save us from the painful ordeal we endured, which lasted for what seemed like a lifetime. None of my friends were ever raped in their houses like we were because my friend's mothers were home. Not to mention the fact that we got raped in the middle of the day in our house. Indeed that would've never happened to my friends because their mothers were usually home during the day.

The arrangement of the household was traditional back then on the island. The men worked jobs outside the house while most women were housewives. They stayed at home and looked after their children. If they lived in the country and raised animals as we did, the moms would also care for the animals during the day.

That's one of the reasons why, for a very long time, I blamed my mother for not living at home to ensure our safety. She could have shielded us from the traumatic torture we endured. As a child who suffered through rape, I was hurt and disappointed for not having anyone to protect me. It saddened a part of me even today when I think about my mother's absence. I thought it was the parents' responsibility to keep their kids safe no matter what. For this reason, I feel that if the rape experience has turned me into an overprotective mother, well, so be it. At the very least, I was never an absent mother. I made sure I was always there to protect my children from harm.

When I was a young child, I did not understand domestic violence so I didn't realize that my mother left home to escape an abusive relationship. All I could think about was how my sister and I suffered at the hands of the two rapists. And if there was a mother at home, she could have saved us from the traumatic experience that changed our lives. Nevertheless, I can't speak about my mother's mental state at the time, and I am not going to judge her for the decision she made to save herself. But for me, I could never sleep at night if I wasn't sure if my children were safe. Then again, it could be because of my rape experience that I feel adamant about protecting my children.

The two rapists knew that we had no adult at home to defend us during that particular time of day; they knew that our single father was raising us and that he was at work during the days. They knew we were two young girls home alone, so we were easy prey for predators. Not only were we raped, but they raped us in the middle of the day in our home. We were supposed to be safe in our home; if we can't be safe at home, where can we be safe?

As a child, I couldn't fathom why my mother wasn't living at home with us anymore. The only thing I could think of was that she failed us as a mother. She wasn't there as an adult to protect us from harm when our father was at work. I didn't blame my father because most fathers worked outside the house, so I blamed my mother because most moms were home with their children. But she unknowingly left us vulnerable when she saved herself and moved out several years earlier.

Looking back through my child's eyes, I secretly blamed my sister for being too extroverted and friendly, and this trait invited a couple of rapists into our house. I blamed myself for going after the rapist to help my sister and not being strong enough to fight him off. As I got older and reflected on what I could have done differently, I thought maybe if I bit the rapist who held me as a hostage, perhaps I could have done more to save us. But I was too afraid; I was worried that if I caused him pain by biting him, he would get angry and beat me up. I didn't want to do anything that I wasn't sure would work to fend them off.

After I grew up, I realized that the rape we suffered was not my mother or sister's fault. Rape cannot be anyone else's fault except the perpetrators. When we look for others to shift the blame towards, we are protecting the rapist. I never told my sister that I secretly blamed her after the incident. There was never any mention of our rape after that awful day. It was like that day never existed. It got suppressed by all the other great memories linking my sister and me together. Knowing that we have never had a conversation about the rape, I never got to tell her that I don't blame her for the horrible tragedy that happened to us. I am an adult now, and the only people I blame for the anguish we went through that day are the two rapists.

Rapists who decide to prey on innocent children are like wild animals that lurk in the dark for a chance at their target. They are the kind of predators that are dangerous criminals, and they should be in prison for life. In my opinion, if you don't know how to conduct yourself as a human being, then the answer is simple, maybe you shouldn't be around humans.

How could she be responsible for something that a couple of adult rapists decided to do? She was just a child; none of us asked two rapist adults to stick their nasty body parts inside of us. Nobody wanted to lose control over their own body, and in particular, no child would want anyone to rape them. My sister had no idea anything like this could have ever happened to us in a million years. Now that I know better, I understand there's no way this could have been her fault. But I was a child suffering psychologically and seeking answers to my numerous questions.

Now that I'm no longer a child, I can think with a far more rational mind. I know it would have been more beneficial for me to run down the street and call for help. In my kid's mind at the time, I didn't want to leave my sister unattended and alone with the rapist. I was worried for her, not knowing what he would do to her behind my back; I was desperate to get her away from him.

Another part of the shame I felt from getting raped was that we got gang-raped. I had to deal with the additional humiliation attached to that type of rape. We were programmed to believe that only certain girls get rape, not to mention gang-raped which was extremely bad. It was bad enough for a girl to get raped, but gang-raped was a double shame on the girl.

I don't know where we learned that rape is the victims' fault or where the root of this brainwash came about. We were programmed from an early age to blame the victim of rape; the programming started from such an early age that I don't remember where in my environment I got it. The code of conduct in which you blame and humiliate the victims of rape has been in place for far too long. Now is the time to shift it to the perpetrators where it belongs.

Many of our beliefs and habits are paradigms of our parents and our environment. It is a learned behavior for victims to blame themselves for the rape. We don't remember when the self-blame and shame got downloaded into our subconscious minds.

That could be because much of the programming we received was before the age of seven.

Victim blaming comes with guilt and shame, and shame is why the secret is associated with rape. It seems like there is an expectation that victims of rape, despite their age, should be responsible for ensuring their safety from pedophiles/rapists. I think predators behave as though they cannot control themselves from overpowering and raping individuals; they act as if they don't know any better, like animals that cannot differentiate between right and wrong.

As girls, the message we got from all the information floating around us that became a part of our conditioning was that if we ever got raped, it was our fault, and we should be ashamed to let ourselves be victims of rape. As mentioned earlier, there was shame associated with a girl in Jamaica if one rapist rapes her. But when it's more than one rapist, the street name was called gang-rape, which was even more humiliating for the survivor. A myth that surface was that gang-rape only happens to bad girls who run around with many different men and that those girls were generally very promiscuous. I realized that rape has nothing to do with the victim and everything to do with the perpetrator.

With that myth in mind, you can only imagine the mental struggles we had at such a young age. We were terrified knowing what our community would think of us if someone uncovered our gang-rape secret. The suffering for me was genuinely sad, not only for the physical wounds I suffered but for a lifetime of emotional and psychological scars.

After the rape happened, I was acutely focused on the shame of us getting raped, and the label of being seen as street girls if anyone knew about the ordeal. The anxiety I endured from keeping the secret seemed endless. In my young child's mind at the time, the most important thing I could think of was that I could not let anyone discover this shameful incident; for "our safety," it must remain cloaked beneath the stains of that day's emotional trauma.

The fear of my secret being found out left me no other choice but to keep quiet about the horrific situation because I had to protect our reputation. If anyone found out about our rape, especially about the type of rape we got, the community would perceive us as two bad street girls. We didn't want anyone to think of us as promiscuous girls. The fact is, as far as I knew at the time, bad girls were the only girls who got gang-raped, so I was perplexed about whether or not we were bad girls.

We are programmed to believe that if a girl is promiscuous, she is seen as a "bad girl" and deserves to get raped. This unhealthy perception that the "bad girls" deserved to get gang-raped was accepted. Rape is a criminal offense and should never be tolerated. Even if the girl sleeps around, she does not deserve to get rape. It's as if rape is the punishment a girl has to pay for her promiscuity. It has to be her fault because how dare she sleep around? That is why in many countries, when a sex worker goes missing or when he/she is murdered, that crime gets less compassion from the public than someone who is not a sex worker.

Knowing what happened to my sister and me, I am not quick to judge anyone. We were afraid of being regarded as "bad girls," which would be wrong because we were two young girls who got raped and were not sleeping around. I used my situation to measure someone else's situation. However, I can see how our programming creates our perception, and they can be wrong. Sometimes, we don't know the whole story, we don't know the sex worker story, so who are we to judge? Maybe instead of judging others, we could have a conversation with them and ask them what happened to them.

On the other side of the programming, we get is that a boy who sleeps around is considered a stud, and as such his peers admire him. This double standard means that we do not teach our boys how to be responsible, empathetic members of society. We tell boys that it's normal to continue with bad behavior because "boys will be boys." While girls are ridiculed for sleeping around, boys get compensated for the same behavior. Here is the question, who made up these rules?

When all these types of confusion and terrifying thoughts and emotions were going through my young mind at the time, it was all the more reason to keep quiet. I was afraid of being treated like one of those stereotyped "bad girls" because I wasn't a bad girl; I was a great girl. But in an instant, with no fault of my own, I was suddenly stripped of all my dignity. Even though I didn't tell anyone about the rape, it felt like everyone knew what happened. That's because I knew that it occurred, and I didn't feel the same way about myself as I did before the rape. I suddenly felt like I was nothing because I thought: if someone is treating you like garbage, you must be garbage.

I felt as if anyone could see that I was gang-raped just by looking at me. The confidence I had about myself before the rape was gone, and I felt like I was dead inside for a very long time. Don't get me wrong, I've learned to cover it up very well. I've learned to smile on the outside and pretend to be happy. Children learn at a very young age to pretend that everything is fine while they suffer in silence. I struggled with anxiety because of what happened on that depressing day. It was a long and challenging journey for me to move from a rape victim to a rape survivor. It wasn't an easy task, but I eventually made it to the other side. I am here to tell you that it is possible.

I suffered from the recurring sexual assault nightmare for several years. Despite the traumatic and disrespectful ordeal I was subjected to, I was a good actor. So at home, I managed to remain the same great and responsible girl that I'd always been. But I believe if parents are aware and paying great attention to their children's behavior, they might be able to see it in their eyes. I said you could see it in their eyes because the eyes are the window to the soul, and they don't lie. Although the child might be smiling and laughing, you must realize that that is what children do and they are good at it. However, the eyes will remain sad, hopeless, and ashamed. So here is a cue for parents, you should watch their eyes while smiling and if you say something as simple as "Are you OK?" A sensitive child who is hurting may immediately start to cry, so just by asking that one question, you realize that the child is not OK. When that happens, it could open up a door for you to create an honest conversation with your child.

If someone had said that to me when I was a child suffering from a vicious rape, I don't believe I could have handled it by just saying "yes, I'm OK" with a straight face. I would break down in tears because I was an emotional wreck for a very long time after the rape. I was the oldest child who lived in our home as I mentioned earlier that my older sister wasn't living in our home when the rape happened. She'd come to visit me that day. Being the oldest at home, my father entrusted me with the financial responsibility of budgeting for our weekly groceries.

He gave me a certain amount of cash on the Friday of each week, and it was my duty to determine the grocery store's budget and the amount to be spent separately in the market. I have to say that it was a big responsibility for a young girl, but it didn't bother me; I enjoyed it. I came to realize that it was probably his way of teaching us about money and budgeting.

It certainly helped me learn about money and the importance of a household budget when I became an adult. Besides, taking on those responsibilities enabled my single dad to focus on other necessary issues for his family. We did whatever we could for him to relieve the weight of being a working single parent. I was a very mature and responsible person growing up.

These transferable budgeting skills helped me financially when I became a single mother with three children to raise. In contrast with my father, I had to look after my children with my only source of income. My father, however, had multiple income streams. My father was very proud of his kids; he used to brag to his friends that he had the best children in our neighborhood. How many kids do you know who take pride in going home after school to prepare dinner for their family? We were among these children.

After school, one of us older kids usually prepared dinner for our family, partly because we needed to eat. The biggest reason though was to make sure our single dad didn't have to cook for us after a hard day of work. Instead of him coming home to cook for us, he came home to a home-cooked meal.

Growing up in a single-parent family has its advantages. One advantage for us was that we learned to cook at a very young age. Being able to cook allowed us to help our single father by preparing delicious, healthy meals for our family.

Luckily, our father raised us to be kind, considerate, and compassionate people. These same qualities allow us to feel empathy for our hard-working single dad. We gave our father the support he needed as a single dad to make his life a little easier. Our dad got to live his life as though he had a wife at home to prepare his meals. Not only did we prepare his dinner, but we also made his breakfast in the morning, and he had his lunch to take with him to work. Again, this is just a snapshot of the kind of kids we were.

Although it was challenging for him to be a single father, he was fortunate to have such helpful children; we were always willing to do our best to make his life a little easier. We did it because we loved and cared about our dad. He knew that he raised sympathetic children who cared deeply about him, and he appreciated and loved us sincerely.

I am giving you a glimpse into our childhood home because I want to provide you with a sense of what kind of children we were. Most of us believe that every human has empathy in our hearts, but it awakened me when I came across the two rapists. That was why I was shocked when the second rapist who showed up wasn't there to help us. I had to wonder if the parents of both rapists had raised them to have compassion for others.

We've never had a conversation in our household discussing sexual violation in any form when we were growing up. I don't recall our father ever telling us to blame ourselves or not blame ourselves if we ever got raped. Sexual violence in any form was never a dialogue in our family. One of the reasons parents don't have this conversation with their children could be that parents don't think to prepare children for rape. They don't want to assume that something as evil as rape could ever happen to their babies in a million years.

A discussion about improper touching is a healthy conversation to have in any home with children. It would help if you talked to your children about inappropriate touching and rape. Once you establish a safe space for children to have an open dialogue, they are more likely to speak freely about improper sexual misconduct. When children feel safe, it is more encouraging for them to talk to someone about rape. Children should always be encouraged to tell someone about any sexual assault in any form.

The truth is that young girls get brainwashed into believing the biased and corrupt lesson that regardless of the girl's age, she is responsible for keeping herself safe from rapist predators. If she's not strong enough to defend herself against the rapist and he takes advantage of her, then she should feel ashamed of something beyond her control in which someone did to her. None of this makes any sense. I consistently wonder who came up with these shameful and idiotic rules.

I can't help but wonder, how exactly did we get here? It's such an idiotic way of thinking and this rule has given abusers too many rights and power and they become complacent. They think they are always right because the rules are all stock in their favor. That being the case, how could they possibly be wrong? One of the first things that work for them is knowing the victims will be too ashamed to say anything to anyone. That alone is a confidence booster for them, so they don't have to worry about being found out.

It is mind-boggling to think that two girls, or any child for that matter, can be held accountable for an adult rapist's behavior. How the heck is that possible? These are some of the reasons why those important platforms, like the #MeToo movement encourages dialogue around unwanted sexual behaviors.

I hope that after reading this book, parents will use this opportunity to have the necessary conversation with their children about any inappropriate touching that makes them feel uncomfortable. This movement is not just for you as an adult to free yourself from the stigma and emotional suffering of sexual violence but you can also use it as a way to talk to your children. Tell them that no one can blame them for being a victim of sexual assault.

When I realized the #MeToo movement was finally working to help punish sex offenders for their sexual, predatory behavior, I was delighted to know that it finally happened; their time was up. That is what Oprah Winfrey said, "Time's up," in her speech at the 2018 Golden Globe Award Show. Women who are struggling with sexual harassment in all its forms were ignored for too long. The time has come once and for all for society to make the wrong right.

The day came when women decided to stand united and regain their power. There's a saying that, "Power is in the numbers." This statement is relevant in the #MeToo movement and when you work together as a team, you are more robust and can achieve much more.

The women who were victims of sexual misconduct, supported by some great men, all decided that enough was enough. The synergy of everyone working together gave them the courage and strength to do something about unwanted sexual advances once and for all. The force of this movement has helped remove the shame from the victims, one layer at a time. The small fire that started burning by a few people got bigger and bigger until it became uncontrollable. It triggered the conversation about sexual assault, sexual harassment, and rape everywhere. When all was said and done, a movement was born out of this surreal moment in time. I pray for every woman who died with the shame of rape that got buried with them. I also stand with all the survivors who made it to see the disgraced rapists as they collapsed and fell.

How the Rape Affected My Parenting

Studies show that the emotional trauma experienced by sexual violence doesn't just stop with that assault victim. Unfortunately, it has a domino effect; it may affect the victim's children's development, their coping mechanisms, and even their interpersonal relationships.

The demon of sexual assault can follow the survivors for their entire life, and sometimes it can manifest itself, most unusually, in so many different ways. It may also be apparent that survivors are overly protective of their children because of the chronic fear of the "what if." They are sometimes fearful that their children may suffer the same fate they did, making them highly protective.

Scientific America found that a mother's parenting style can affect the activity of a child's gene. Parents are genetic engineers because they shape the genetics of their children. The study of Epigenetics shows that the environment controls Biology; this means that a significant amount of responsibility is on the parents. The mother's environment influences the gene during the child's development in the womb. If the mother is fearful or stressed, the unborn child will experience those same emotions.

Some adults who are stressed and depressed don't understand why they feel those emotions. Dr. Bruce Lipton, an American developmental biologist, is notable for his views on epigenetics. He said, "The mother is the headstone in nature because she has to prepare the child biologically, even before it's born, to survive in the environment where she lives." My childhood rape caused RTS (Rape Trauma Syndrome) to be a part of my environment. Epigenetics says these emotions don't stop with me but are passed down to my children.

It's unfortunate for children, especially the first generation of somebody who has had a traumatic encounter. The paranoia of raising children from fear can make them socially awkward; it can cause anxiety disorder and numerous other mental and social issues.

After my husband left our family, I became a single mother of three young children, one son and two daughters. My son had just turned thirteen, my eldest daughter was ten, and my youngest was only seven years old when he left.

I never got remarried, and I dedicated all my attention to raising my children. I will admit that I was always fearful for their safety, which played a significant role in their upbringing. Raising my kids was my number one priority in life, and the last thing I wanted to do was invite a male into their life who wasn't their biological father. For that reason, I decided against getting remarried.

The thought of remarrying a new husband to live with me and my young children triggered my childhood rape experience. I was afraid for my children's safety, primarily because of being frozen in the past. I didn't want my children to feel unsafe or uncomfortable in the home. I analyze every situation that involves them, and I tried my best to keep them from living with the trauma of rape like I had to live with my entire life.

Don't get me wrong, I know that most men are good people, but there's a small percentage of bad guys out there. And the last thing I wanted to do was take my chances and sequentially marry one of the bad guys. So I decided against it and concentrated on bringing up my children as a single mother.

I gave my children the protection that I would have wanted from my mother when I was a child on the day of the rape. But the difference was that when the rape occurred, my mother was no longer living in our home. I agree that some of the decisions I made when I raised my children were from fear because of my rape experience. But in my mind, I did it to keep my children safe and for my peace of mind.

I became very good at analyzing every situation having to do with my children; I would see if any loopholes exist in each circumstance as I try to ensure safety. This approach allowed me to feel at ease when making certain decisions, specifically those that have to do with my children. I now know that most of my parenting decisions were essentially rape protection decisions, disguised as security.

My rape experience had me so frightened for my children's safety that I would see danger even when there was none. I never told them how consumed I was about their safety, afraid that someone might want to rape them. I didn't want them to walk around feeling paranoid out of their wits. That's why I kept the gravity of my fear from them.

I kept the deep-seated reason for my fear to myself; I didn't want my kids to know why I felt the way I did. All they knew was that I was looking out for their best interests because I loved them. That was true, but there was more to my paranoia; I was overly cautious because of the anxiety of being raped.

I essentially became a puppet on a string. I was the puppet, and the string was the chronic fear from my rape. The memories of my shocking rape were a constant trigger for me in several areas of my life. My children had no idea that I was terrified for their welfare and, even as an adult, Rape Trauma Syndrome is a constant struggle.

I did everything I could to prevent them from suffering from the same fate as I did. As a mother, I provided them with the safety that I wish I had from my mother. My only problem was that I used my own rape experience as my guide in raising them. I provided my children with the level of protection that would hinder a rapist from raping them in our home.

My rape ordeal programmed me to raise my kids out of fear. Even though I was able to protect them from sexual predators, I know that I based many of my decisions on rape avoidance. I guess in the end I've ensured the level of security around them the best way I knew how. It may not have been the most appropriate way to raise them, but it was better than nothing.

Looking back, I know I've probably overreacted in some cases, but I've never been an absent parent. I was a hands-on parent, my ears were on, and my eyes were on in every way possible. Everything I did was all in the name of protecting my kids from harm.

In my heart, I believe that I have given my kids enough protection from any form of sexual abuse in their childhood. But it's a real shame that my rape anxiety caused my children to miss out on many childhood fun with their friends. I can admit that numerous activities I told them they could not attend were decisions based on my fear and bias.

That said, one of the things that were very difficult for me to bring myself to allow my children to do with their friends was sleepovers. I found it very challenging to give them consent to have sleepovers at their friends' homes. When they were teenagers, maybe I allowed it once or twice, but I had to investigate the host home's parents before granting my permission. After doing my homework and being satisfied with what I found out, I would only allow a sleepover. These were some of the times when I was thrilled that I was the only parent who made all the parental decisions for my children. It was great that I didn't have a spouse to challenge and argue with my choices. My ex-husband was not involved in their upbringing, so I became the sole decision-maker in our family.

When I had to make my decision, I asked many questions, and based on the answers I received, it helped with having clarity about the sleepover. And even when I agreed to the sleepover, it didn't mean I wasn't worried about my kids' safety. However, I took some risks to make them feel "normal" and happy, and to the best of my knowledge, most of the decisions I made paid off.

The few times I succumbed to the slumber party pressure from them I realized that they desperately wanted to fit in with their slumber party friends. Although I often suffered from the anguish of the "what if," I wanted them to have some fun and stop complaining about my choices. I felt the fear, but I did it regardless. It allowed them to feel happy, pleased, and normal.

I never told them the real reason they weren't allowed to do sleepovers and many other children's activities. It was my need to protect them from the evil I knew firsthand existed in the world. I knew that evil lurked among us because I experienced this evil when I was a child.

In theory, children are so innocent and kind, they tend to look at everyone as good people just like themselves. They don't understand how insensitive, selfish and cruel some adults can be, and our job is to shield them from those cruel ones.

I know most people are good, but my rape experience didn't even allow me to consider this to be true. And the reason is that it's tough to differentiate the good guys from the bad guys just by looking at them.

As mentioned, my childhood rape experience has dictated most of the decisions I've made in my life. It was the reason I was so overprotective of my children, I didn't want the same thing that happened to my sister and me to happen to anybody else, let alone my children. I didn't want them to go through such a horrible and frightening situation. The following is an example of one of my fearful parenting dilemmas.

My youngest daughter once attended a French immersion school outside the area where we lived at the time. The school bus did not want to pick her up and drop her off because they said it was outside their school schedule section. Due to that, I would drive her to and from school.

As a result of traffic and sometimes bad Canadian weather, I was sometimes late to pick her up from school. It got a little frightening when I went to pick her up one evening after school and she was standing by the side of the street. She was standing in the cold for quite a long while, waiting for me to get her. That was when I told her to ask her father for a key to his house so she could wait for me in a safe and warm environment.

Her dad, my ex-husband, lived near the school our daughter attended, so it would be safe for her to walk to his home after school. She didn't have to walk by herself as some of her school friends lived close by; they could easily walk together. I was disappointed when she asked her dad for a key to his house, and he told her that he would have to think about it. He eventually suggested that she could go to his sister's house instead of his home.

My ex-husband's sister lived a little further away from the school, but she was still within walking distance. Her father lived closer to the school than her aunt, still, he suggested that she go to his sister's after school. Maybe it would have been okay if I wasn't looking at it through the experience of my rape lenses.

At this point, the distance was not my only concern; I was very uncomfortable with this suggestion. Let me explain why. I was more at ease with the idea that my daughter is staying at her father's house after school rather than her aunt's house. After examining her aunt's home environment, I looked at the people who lived in that house and how well I knew these people. The rape experience started to show me all the things that could go wrong with this idea.

Not only did her aunt live farther away from the school than her dad did, but I wasn't exactly familiar with her aunt's husband. Hence, my paranoia immediately led me to think through every possible scenario that could go wrong. What if my daughter showed up at the house to wait for me after school and her aunt wasn't home, but her husband was alone in the house? It would leave my little girl vulnerable and alone with a man I hardly knew. If something were to happen to her, there would be no one there to protect her, just like I had no one to defend me when I got raped. I was petrified to agree to that suggestion, and I was disappointed that her father refused to give his daughter a key to his house.

Make no mistake, I had no reason to believe that her aunt's husband was not a good man; he was probably a decent human being but my paranoia had nothing to do with the husband of my daughter's aunt. It had everything to do with my rape trauma.

The traumatic experience of rape had remained front and center in my subconscious mind, and it kept holding me hostage and forcing me to parent from an anxious space. My fear showed me all the "what ifs" that could go wrong in every situation that I could not control. Once an issue was totally out of my control, I would start panicking.

Her dad's refusal to give her the key to his house triggered my panic attack. I knew it wasn't safe for her to wait by the side of the road, and the thought of her going to her aunt's house scared me. But I had to decide what she should do if I ran a little late to get her after school. After careful consideration, I had no other choice at the time but to tell my daughter it was okay to go to her aunt's house if I was running late.

One day it happened, I was late to pick her up, and she had to walk to her aunt's house. It occurred only once, and it was a bad experience for her. After school, one cold and snowy winter day, my daughter walked to her aunt's house only to realize that there was nobody at home to let her in. You can imagine how hurt and angry I was when I found out about the situation, knowing that if only she had the key to her father's house she could have easily waited for me there. That way, she'd be safe from harm, and she wouldn't have to stay in the cold.

Her dad worked the afternoon shift, so naturally, she would be home by herself. But I would feel more comfortable if she were alone at her dad's house than alone on the cold street corner. She'd be safe in her dad's house because she knew to lock the door behind her and not let anybody inside. After discovering there was no one at her aunt's place, she returned to the spot on the street where I usually pick her up after school. I was pretty upset that her father wouldn't give his daughter the key to his house in the name of safety.

I felt a little guilty that I was more at ease in the depths of my heart knowing that there was no one in her aunt's house to receive her. Deep down, I somehow preferred that outcome rather than her aunt's husband being alone with my little girl.

It's just an example of how the two rapists' choice to rape us that day has influenced my way of thinking and making decisions. It caused me to be overly cautious. I have often wondered how I would have been as a parent had I not experienced the trauma of rape. I suppose I'll never find out. The decision those two cruel rapists made that day has changed my life and certainly impacted how I raised my children.

My innocent daughter did not know I preferred that no one was in her aunt's house on that cold and snowy day.

Since her aunt wasn't going to be there, it was better to know that there was no one in the house as far as I was concerned.

Children trust everyone around them. Because they are at a lower brainwave frequency than adults, they cannot consciously analyze and see the danger the way adults can. I believe children are closer to God than adults, therefore, they only see kindness in the world around them. I was one of those children who were incapable of analyzing the situation my sister and I were in the day we got raped. I now know, as an adult, that I should have run down the street and sought help. In addition, when the second rapist showed up, I thought he would help us. I didn't know he was there to help his friend and himself.

As I mentioned, kids can only see everybody as good. Children don't know that some adults are predators who target kids and will hurt them in some of the most horrific ways imaginable. For this reason, the ball is in our court as parents. We must do our best to protect our kids from adults with twisted minds. And sometimes you will be regarded as overprotective, well, that's okay. None of my children have gotten molested or raped. I am not saying that I did the right thing by bringing up my children from my rape fears, but it was all I knew at the time.

My children are adults now, and they are all independent entrepreneurs who not only provide for their well-being but provide jobs for others. Most of the time, children will live what they learn. I'm an independent individual who has worked for myself most of my life. I raised my children alone, and all they know is that their mother worked for herself. That said, I'm assuming I didn't do half a lousy job influencing them on the career part. I might have to write another book to tell you if the rape trauma has found its way into the next generations and influenced them socially.

If you are wondering how their social life is working out for them, or should you wish to know more about that, please let me know in your feedback.

Predators have no idea or care to know that the sexual assault they exercised and forgotten about has harmed and tarnished the survivor's life forever. And sometimes, the suffering and fear don't end with that individual. No, it is like a vine that will grow and thrive; and just like a vine, with a suitable environment, the fear and anxiety can live for many generations.

Having lived through the long-term impacts of sexual assault, I can tell you that it influenced the way I brought up my children. My paranoia deprived them of having a fun-filled childhood. Instead, they had a fear-based one. It was my responsibility as a parent to advocate for my children against the "big bad wolves" of child sexual predators. I took my parenting responsibilities very seriously. And, I did it my way to shield them from harm.

My way was the best way I knew how. I hope my children realize that whatever happens, I did my best to make sure they could escape the nightmare of being raped as children. That is a nightmare they would have to carry with them for the rest of their lives, and the attachments accompanying rape are shame and guilt.

I was that protective mother who drove her children everywhere they needed to go. I had the luxury of having flextime because I was self-employed. For some reason, my professional life blossomed, I didn't allow the trauma of rape to affect how I ran my business, and I managed to pass the entrepreneurial spirit down to all my children. I am not a psychologist, so I can't speak on why that is the case. But it just so happens that they are all self-employed.

My children took public transportation a few times in their lives; this was when there was no other choice. When it happened, however, I was very paranoid and concerned for their safety. I had thoughts like "what if" someone follows them off the bus and violates them? Or when they wait for the bus at the bus stop, "what if" someone tries to restrain them?

I sometimes would imagine my daughters being restrained with nobody to help them. I would see a play-by-play scene from my rape experienced happening to them. The horrific images lodged on the recorder in my subconscious mind were readily accessible. I would relive my experience happening to my kids, and there was no one there to help them. I would imagine them being as helpless as I was. I often had to convince myself to snap out of it, to get over it, but it was a constant battle.

I remember how terrified I was when my sister and I needed somebody to help us, and even now when I think about that horrible day, I can still feel those awful emotions I felt that day. I can attest to the level of fear when you seek help and no one comes to the rescue. It is sometimes still very fresh in my memory, especially when an experience triggers it. It can still feel like it had just happened yesterday.

One shocking thing for me was that he wasn't there to help us when someone finally came along. He helped his rapist friend and helped himself instead. He teamed up with the first rapist and they both raped us. When we cried and pleaded with them to let us go, they did not care for us, and our cries fell on deaf ears.

We were completely at their mercy, and all we could do was beg them to have a heart and have pity on us. But they were not going to have any of this because we meant nothing to them. Essentially, it was going to be their way or no way. Their action devastated me, and the rape trauma changed the trajectory of my life. However, I still believe, and I want to take this time to communicate to you, that most people in the world are good people.

It Was Called Battery

There was a derogatory name associated with sexual assault (rape) involving more than one rapist. An example of this would be the kind of rape that happened to my sister and me. When a girl was raped by more than one rapist during the same initial rape act, in Jamaica, the street name of that gang rape was called a battery.

When a girl experiences a battery rape, she would be looked down- on and seen as a loose or bad girl in most cases. This culture stuck with me because not only were we raped, we were gang-raped, and the gang-rape aspect has an added emotional stigma attached to the rape.

Now that we got raped or gang-banged, there was an added new level of shame on us. Generally speaking, men who commit this kind of rape were admired a little by their peers. Some of them even go as far as to brag about the battery they performed on certain girls, and their peers would be eager to hear all the details. At the same time, the women who had to endure the act would be considered bad, promiscuous girls.

Essentially, the girl would be labeled as a "not-so-nice girl." She is not the kind of woman an honest man would want to marry. Can you believe that? This social construct manipulates others into believing that the girl who got raped deserves punishment for being raped. It is not her fault for what happened to her, but she doesn't deserve to have a decent man marrying her.

This same gang-rape act in some other parts of the world is called gang-bang. No matter what the action was labeled as, the shame was on the girl who was defeated and raped. Unfortunately, the rapist men are left with no shame and they can brag about the rape without any consequence.

Take a look at this scenario: A few men choose to control and rape a woman by restraining her with strong, masculine, and physical strength. That rape act essentially takes away her right to her own body; it is her body, but she has no say in what should or should not happen to her body. The rapists took it over, and she got removed from making any choice concerning her physical well-being. However, society feels it deem to make this her fault, and the rapist used this kind of trickery to hide behind their rape crime. This type of behavior by rape attackers happens in many cultures all over the world.

First, they found a way to manipulate the victim into believing the rape is supposed to be their fault, and expect the girl to feel disgraced; the ability to comprehend this has escaped me. How does that make any sense? It is what some would call fake news. It does not matter how they spin this scenario and look at it, it does not make any logical sense. How can they blame a woman, let alone a child, who does not have the physical strength to fight off one or two strong male rapists? It is not going to happen; it is unlikely that she will be successful.

Where does the logic rest in that situation? The attacker gets to walk around and brag about what they have done to women and girls. They are allowed to brag to their friends without being judged for the rape crime. They take great pride in the rape they have committed, and their friends will consider them macho or stud. How sick does one have to be not to realize the level of evil in this act?

Suppose these rapists begin to boast to their friends about the battery rape they were involved in, the girls would have to go into hiding due to the extra shame and guilt stacked up against them. Women do not want to talk about rape to anybody for fear of being labeled bad, promiscuous girls. However, the rapist can speak freely, and sometimes they even inflate the details about their performance during the rape so that they appear more macho to their friends.

The mindset of many rapists is to disrespect and humiliate their victims. As far as we were concerned, that was probably a part of their plan. This could be true because not only were we violated, we also got held against our will and were forced to watch each other's humiliation and torture as we got gang-raped by both rapists.

The humiliation I felt from the trauma of that rape was horrifying. Nevertheless, the psychological trauma of watching my sister and not being able to do anything about it was awful. I felt embarrassed for her and myself. At the same time, I was there waiting and wondering about my fate. I suppose they wanted to display their power and control over two children. They must have felt very robust to be able to overpower and rape children.

The Rapists' Reputation

The first rapist:
The first rapist who dragged my sister into the house was the father of many children in our community. He had children with numerous young schoolgirls in our area. And there were rumors on the street that he had raped several of these young girls with whom he had children.

Naturally, he would deny the rape happened and dismiss the child as his which assassinates the girl's characters. When he rejects the children, it's a double shame on the girls because now she is perceived as a loose girl who sleeps around and has no clue who her child's father is. I suppose by admitting the children were his, he would have to pay child support, so he took the easy and selfish way out by denying the children were his.

Despite the undesirable situation to which he subjected those young girls, he would also say negative things about them. Things like there was no way he would let anyone see him with such a low-class girl. I'm sure you must be wondering who exactly is the low-class person here. He also disrespected some of the girls he raped by calling them ugly. He would use many other unflattering descriptive words to discredit girls and push them further into hiding. When this happens the girls end up suffering alone in silence.

You can imagine the impact this has on a young girl's self-esteem, especially if she is pregnant due to her rape. If this girl is raped and got pregnant following the rape, the girl suffered twice for something she had no control over. If this was what he did to young girls, he should be ashamed of himself for raping children and then acting superior to them.

Based on what he did to my sister and me, I can't say I doubt the rumors. I believe he did rape those girls and impregnated them. How can a rapist find himself in a class superior to that of the innocent girls he raped? You have to be delusional to have this sort of mindset in the first place. Some of these young mothers have to drop out of school to become full-time moms, and some of them were children themselves.

Furthermore, while there was a rumor in our district that he was a rapist, he would dismiss it, and there was never any consequence for his criminal behavior. Another way he could escape punishment was that nobody had ever reported him to the police, as far as I know. The girls were usually too ashamed to say anything about the rape. Girls sometimes remain silent because they would most likely be called promiscuous instead of victims, and they don't want to carry that additional shame.

I was too young to conceptualize some of the whispers circulating about that particular rapist at the time. And although many adults were aware of his actions, nobody did anything to protect the young girls in our district from him. I don't know whether it was because everybody in our community knew him and his family. Additionally, some of the victims may have even been his relatives.

I am not sure if that was the case why the victims never reported him to the police, but if it were, the last thing they would want to do would be to send one of their relatives to jail for rape. I don't understand why he wasn't reported to the police by the parents of some of the girls with whom he had children. They never felt the need to go to the police. Looking back now, maybe the parents all thought their daughters were "bad girls." I know I didn't say anything to anyone because I was too humiliated to admit I got raped. Moreover, I had no idea how to turn someone over to the police. You have to understand that I was a child when he raped me.

The silence around his rape secret confirms that it probably had something to do with the belief around rape and the victims of rape in that era. At that period in time, it appeared that the culture surrounding rape and sexual exploitation of children was not as severely taboo as it is today. They may not have understood how traumatic rape was to anybody, let alone a young child. They had no understanding of Rape Trauma Syndrome and how it disrupts physical, emotional, and cognitive functions.

They had no idea of the impact rape has on survivors of rape because not even the survivors could explain their suffering. Young girls are usually incapable of verbalizing their deeper emotions, therefore they would suffer in silence.

When the rapist denied the babies he made from raping those girls, it made them look like they were sleeping around. This is devastating for a decent young girl's self-worth to be viewed as promiscuous. It made her out to be someone who was sleeping with many different men, and because of that, they honestly didn't know which one of them was the father of the child. That in itself is abusive towards girls.

The vulnerable girls were walking with their heads hanging in shame while the rapist re-victimized them by lying about them. Not only that, but the baby is a constant reminder of that rape. As the victim goes through all the confusion and embarrassment, the sex predator bravely seeks his next victim.

Later when I became an adult, I looked back at all the adults who used to whisper that he raped young girls and impregnated them. When I looked back at the tone around child rape at the time, I can honestly say that I can't remember when any of those adults became angry about these sex predators being allowed to roam our streets freely.

The adults were very naive about the length he would go to rape the girls. They had no idea that he would even go inside the girl's house if he had to. He would do whatever it take to perform his rape acts. If the girl can't be safe in her home, where can she be safe? He had many children by many different girls, and the ones he acknowledged as his children, he acted as if he was having a relationship with the young girls. He was very cunning and knew precisely how to manipulate the situation.

He would perform his act after the parents realized that their daughters were pregnant. Now, when I look back at his crafty behavior, I come to realize that he was a real con artist who knew exactly how to cover his tracks.

Some of the girls told their parents that he had raped them and made them pregnant, but the parents never really did anything about it. If they reported him to the police, I would have heard about it because the people in our community would talk. This talk would including whether or not he got arrested for rape. As aforementioned, everyone in our district would know about it because he was a local celebrity.

I was a young girl when a lot of the chatter about him raping schoolgirls in our community started surfacing, but I was unaware of the depth of his sexual assault stories at the time. Children are sometimes the last to know about adult secrets. For the most part, adults would not speak about rape and sex in general in the presence of children. The word sex was a taboo subject to discuss in front of children.

As far as I know, I don't remember anyone ever pressing rape charges against the rapist for his criminal behavior. The adults in our community would only whisper about him behind closed doors.

I can only imagine that he denied raping the young girls he impregnated to their parents. Even if he claimed that the act was consensual between him and the girls, he should still be in trouble with the law if that was his defense. That's because the girls were minors, and minors cannot give sexual consent. So why was he having a sexual relationship with a minor? That is because he was a pedophile and a rapist.

In reality, it is tough for a woman to come forward in the first place to talk about rape and any sexual violence. And it is three or four times as hard for a young girl to have the courage to tell somebody about a sexual assault she experienced. That is if she eventually builds up the nerve to tell someone. Most of the time the secret got revealed because the girl gets pregnant due to the rape.

It would be difficult for her if she came forward and told her story about what happened to her, only for the rapist to turn around and deny it happened. Although the rape occurred, it becomes his word against hers if he denies it. Then, the cruel manipulating adult rapist would twist and fix the story to help himself out of the situation.

If you ever wondered how a child could consent to have sexual relations with an adult, you are not alone; I wondered about that myself. I noticed how his sexual violation affected some of the girls he turned into young mothers in our community. You can visually see the changes in some of these girls' physical appearance. They seemed wounded, they lost their self-esteem and dignity. Some even started acting out of control.

The girls were crying out for psychological help; some of them had even become promiscuous. And some girls ended up having two or three children before the age of twenty. After the first baby with the rapist, some of the girls were never the same. Some girls became self-destructive after having babies with the rapist.

The rape they experienced, thanks to the rapist, changed the path they were on. Some of these vulnerable young girls he violated did not know what to do with the shame and the hurt they felt. The rape they experienced drove them to rebel, so they started sleeping around with different men. And, sad to say, sometimes the men were as old as their fathers.

Of course, we never told anyone about what he did to us, so I can imagine how many other girls suffered by him raping them and kept quiet about it too. I got raped as a child, and I just developed the courage to speak about what happened to me and my sister. If I were to disclose the location in Jamaica where the rape occurred, we might be able to start our #MeToo movement in our district.

I don't want to mention their names, but whenever anyone from our district reads about our story, they will pinpoint who they are, especially the first rapist. The second rapist will be a little more challenging to identify by the people in my neighborhood.

I know for sure that we were not his only victims, and neither were we his last. He continued to rape young girls under the age of consent, and he continued to get away with it. He eventually migrated to live in the United States of America, having no criminal records whatsoever.

As far as I know, his life was never tarnished in any way with any rape crime in Jamaica. Unfortunately, I can't say the same for the girls he raped. Girls who experience rape have to live with their label of either victims or survivors of rape in perpetuity.

While writing this book, I heard that he had moved back from the United States to live in Jamaica in the same family home he lived in when he raped us. I also heard that he had reunited with some of his now-adult children that he denied when they were babies. I understood that he apologized to some of his children for not being there as a dad.

Now that he is back and is living in the same community, I can only hope that he is too old now to continue on his usual rape path. I empathize with all of his victims and hope for the young girls' safety in the community.

The second rapist:
The second rapist's father was a friend of my father. The second rapist was the one who restrained me and had me watch the first rapist rape my sister. At that time, I wasn't aware that I was waiting to be gang-raped by both of them.

He was known for being a gambler and for getting into fights. Some people in the district were afraid of him because he had a bad temper. He usually walked around with a knife and was not afraid to use it.

He had been in several physical fights throughout the years. A few years after we got raped, he got into a fight with someone at one of his gambling games. He stabbed his gambling opponent and received a prison sentence for his actions. We kept our rape a secret so he was never punished for raping us. I don't know if we were his first rape victims or not; this is because I'd never heard of him being a rapist.

I feel in my heart that he must have committed rape acts before he raped us. I concluded that because he didn't hesitate to holding me against my will and participated in raping us. He restrained me until his friend raped my sister and he didn't mind waiting for his turn. In addition, he wasn't bothered by the hurt they both inflicted on us as he didn't hesitate to pass me off to his rapist friend. He handed me over to his friend like a piece of meat to be raped by the first rapist who had just finished raping my sister. His sadistic mindset prevented him from having any problems taking his rape turn on us.

I blocked out some of the horrific details from the rape because it is emotionally draining for me to go back to that place and time. I remember that he wasn't the first one to rape me, but he was the one who restrained me and had me watch the rape of my sister.

I remember that he held me for what seemed like forever until his rapist friend was through with my sister. The second rapist didn't rape me initially, and I wondered if he possibly thought that I was too young, short, and skinny. I was a very skinny kid, and I'm not trying to give him any credit. I just wondered why he didn't feel the need to rape me when he had me restrained.

He eventually raped me after his friend stopped tearing me into pieces. I suppose after he noticed that I was still alive, he had no problem taking his turn to rape what was remaining of me. This happened, as you well know, after the first rapist raped my sister; I still don't know the real reason he held me without raping me. It's hard to speculate about his cause for not raping me initially because he eventually still ended up raping me.

I remained in the same community for several years after the rape, and I never heard anything about the second rapist raping anyone else. But you never know because girls won't easily discuss being rape victims. He had no problem gang-raping my sister and me that day so what would prevent him from raping others? I believe he is more guilty than his friend because of the friendship his father had with my father.

How It Affected My Well-being

The rape of my sister and me changed our lives forever. That gruesome day is a topic that was never up for discussion when we got together as siblings. We talked about everything we can remember that happened when we were children, but we never discussed the rape topic. Since the day it happened, my sister and I never spoke about the rape to each other or anyone else. Understandably, we were two frightened young sisters at the time of the rape. But for some reason, we knew enough about the level of shame associated with rape to keep it a secret. We were so scared and embarrassed that we became numbed about the reality of its existence. So, she and I have never faced the facts of the rape, and we have never spoken about it since that day. I was perplexed as to what we might have done that led them into wanting to hurt us so badly.

It was difficult for me to process the trauma of the rape, let alone the shock of the overall experience I underwent. Everything happened so fast without any warning whatsoever. I tried to make some sense of it, but that only drove me into even more profound confusion. I suffered from nightmares and flashbacks of the incident for several years.

The flashbacks appeared very real when they happened. It was as if I relived the ordeal many times over. My experience of reliving the incident when the flashback came is because thoughts are attached to whatever emotion it represents. Suppose you are thinking about a joyous occasion in your life, you will create and relive that event's emotional experience when you think about it.

The suffering is prolonged if your thoughts are about an unpleasant time in your life. That is why people who suffer from depression are encouraged to do meditation and stay in the present moment. My flashback caused me to replay the event with the same painful emotions I suffered. Every time I played the tape of that day, I would experience the trauma of the rape. In essence, I played that tape for many years; I didn't know how not to play the tape. For quite a long time, I couldn't get it out of my mind. The sudden shock of the rape trauma instantly lodged itself into my subconscious mind. As scientists say, we use only five percent of our conscious mind, ninety-five percent of the time we are operating from our subconscious mind.

And given that our subconscious minds are habitual records of past experiences, for many years, I continued replaying the fear and anxiety that sabotaged my life in various ways. It limited the strength of my inner being and left me in a weak and victimized mentality.

The anxiety I felt was from pressing the replay button of the memory recorded in my mind that terrible day. The unpleasant memories in my subconscious mind were readily accessible. The constant rewind of the incident reminded me of how humiliated, violated, helpless, and mentally confused I felt. Although I was powerless as a child when the rape happened, replaying those memories kept me in the same vulnerable state as an adult for a very long time.

The worst part of it was that I didn't feel like I could trust anyone with the secret. I couldn't even speak to my best friend about what happened to us because I was too ashamed and afraid of being judged. Therefore, I wasn't comfortable enough to talk to anyone about my feelings. I kept all the painful emotions I was feeling to myself. The only thing I knew how to do very well was how to push the play button in my subconscious mind. I played that vicious tape constantly. I didn't say anything about the rape to anyone; I just kept playing the tape.

I went through severe paranoia, depression, and anxiety following the shocking rape trauma. I contemplated running away from my community at one point so that I wouldn't have to see those rapists ever again. But the more I thought about it, the more I realized I wouldn't know where to go. So that idea quickly disappeared from my mind.

I can tell you from my experience that depression in children is far worse than when an adult is suffering from depression. I said this because the adult can seek help for their illness, but the child will continue to suffer in silence as they are less likely to know where to turn for help. It is also hard for the child to explain what they are feeling, let alone seek help. It is especially tough when shame is the essence of the anxiety and depression they are having.

I experienced depression after the rape took a toll on my psyche. Many unpleasant and scary thoughts will go through a young child's mind when they are depressed. The worst part is that some young people commit suicide without anyone ever noticing that they needed help.

Several situations can cause a young person to feel depressed and have suicidal thoughts. It can happen if they endure any psychological distress and don't have the emotional support they need. One example of this is when a child suffers from Rape Trauma Syndrome; they are usually alone with their thoughts. Some may think that suicide is the only way to end their pain. Children and even many adults are not aware that they can control when to play the tape. It is not an easy process; it takes a total mind shift to recognize when the tape is on the play button. It took me a long time to realize that I don't play the recording when I am in a state of consciousness.

When a child is in the developmental stages, they are usually dealing with the growing pain of puberty. If he/she has to go through the added pain and stress of rape trauma, that combination can have an overwhelming effect on their mind. Sadly, most of the time the child will deal with rape trauma alone because of the shame associated with rape.

For a very long time after the rape happened, I felt dirty and disgusting physically. The embarrassment and the stigma attached to rape were daunting for me. The burden to keep it a secret because of victim shaming was hard to bear, and it left me feeling unwell, sad, and weak-minded. I didn't want to be perceived negatively by my peers, so my soul shrank like a flower sleeping at night; I folded inward. I gazed at the world from behind that glass, and I was suspicious of everyone; I knew for sure I couldn't trust anyone with the secret. The horror of anyone noticing a difference in my personality scared me, which intensified my anxiety and depression.

Those are some of the reasons that contribute to why victims of rape keep quiet about the assaults. Although I had my family who would be super supportive if they knew about it, I was too ashamed to tell them, so I didn't. Instead, I kept the secret to myself; That decision caused me to live like I was in this world all by myself. It was like I had no one and nowhere to turn. I felt alone and isolated even from my own family.

I was like a walking dead. Until recently, I realized I've been suffering from Rape Trauma Syndrome. I was thrilled to learn that my suffering had a name and that I wasn't the only victim of rape who was suffering from this. Rape Trauma Syndrome has some of the same charismatics of post-traumatic stress disorder (PTSD) suffered by some combat veterans.

Studies show that rape survivors experience similar symptoms when measured physically, behavioral, and psychologically.

An article from the University of St Louis said, *"Rape Trauma Syndrome or {RTS) is related to post-traumatic stress disorder. However, it is more specific to sexual assault. RTS describes trauma symptoms, including disruptions to normal physical, emotional, cognitive and interpersonal behavior."*

The study shows that *"some major symptoms of RTS are:*

1. *Re-Experiencing the Trauma: Rape victims may experience recurrent nightmares about the rape, flashbacks, or may have an inability to stop remembering the rape.*
2. *Social Withdrawal: This symptom has been called 'psychic numbing' and involves not experiencing any feelings.*
3. *Avoidance Behaviors and Actions: Victims may desire to avoid any feelings or thoughts that might recall to the mind events about the rape.*
4. *Increased Physiological Arousal Characteristics: This symptom is like an exaggerated startle response, hyper-vigilance, sleep disorders, or difficulty concentrating.*
5. *Although each individual's experience is unique, people experiencing Rape Trauma Syndrome often process their trauma in a series of stages."*

The article said, *"The major acute stages of Rape Trauma Syndrome (RTS) critical stage can begin days or weeks after a sexual assault. It can generally last for a few days and a few weeks to years of suffering. Often, victims begin experiencing an intense degree of symptoms after the initial shock of an assault has worn off. Symptoms at this stage may include:*

1. *Diminished alertness or hyper-alertness*
2. *Paralyzing anxiety*
3. *Disorganized thought content*
4. *The obsession with washing or cleaning themselves*
5. *Nausea and vomiting*
6. *Numbness*
7. *Confusion about everyday life*
8. *Dulled sensory, affective, and memory functions*
9. *Thoughts of and increased risk of suicide.*
10. *Acute sensitivity to the reaction of other people."*

My nightmares after the rape lasted for what seemed like forever. I suffered from many of the symptoms listed above. I essentially found myself living a double life. On the outside, I would show my teeth so it would appear as though I was happy and smiling joyfully. But on the inside, I was drowning with shame, guilt, and blame; I blamed myself and some family members for the rape. My perception shifted the responsibility from the two pedophiles' to a few innocent individuals who have nothing to do with the rape. But you have to understand the mindset of a child hurting and grasping at a straw. I would do whatever it took to eliminate the emotional turmoil I was going through at that time. For a long time, I blamed my mother for not protecting her children and my sister for being too friendly.

After I suffered from the trauma in silence for several years, I essentially buried it in my subconscious mind and tried to move past it. I learned how to mask it and continue living my life to appear as if the rape had never happened. I eventually stopped thinking about it as an obsession. Nevertheless, the effect of the sexual violation hitched itself in my subconscious mind forever. It dictates how I create and navigate my way through life on numerous levels, particularly my decision-making.

Consciously, I would try my best not to let that bad experience negatively control and direct my everyday life. However, it steers my decisions in many ways, and it never really goes away totally. I am still concerned for my safety and my loved ones sometimes. Plus, to this day, I'm usually cautious of my surroundings. I am fully aware now that the bad experience we suffered that day at the hands of both rapists is only a part of my story. I know that it doesn't define who I am as a person, but I will always be cautious of whom I let into my circle, and I don't trust people as easily.

That experience has become a part of my journey; it is one of my many stories while I am here in this earth school. I have accepted it as one of my many stories. I try not to think about it often; I placed it in the back of my mind as I continue to move forward. It will never disappear from my memory totally, but I learned how to control the tape and the volume as well. I can recognize those thoughts when they try to manipulate my decisions. My viewpoint towards it changed, and that allowed us to co-exist together. I am no longer afraid to own it and its position in my life. That said, I can tell you that the survivors of rape will never forget that they got raped, but I don't think serial rapists care to remember their victims. For me, I don't live in that constant "fight or flight mode anymore." However, the psychological trauma reminds me from time to time to be careful of my surroundings.

As a child living in Jamaica when the rape occurred, I never knew anything about counselors or therapists to assist individuals suffering from trauma. I didn't get any support after my rape, which is very sad because I would have learned that neither my sister nor I was responsible for the rape. I would realize earlier in my life that we didn't do anything wrong and that it was not our fault. It was two adult male rapists who decided it was a good idea to rape children.

Of course, I was also a child when it happened, and for me to see a therapist, I would have to pay for that service. That being the case, I would have to tell someone about the rape. Talking to my dad about our rape was not an option for me. There was too much humiliation attached to the rape we suffered, making it difficult to speak to anyone about that secret. So with this in mind, it would be hard for me to get help.

Essentially, my father would have to take me to see the counselor, and for him to do that, I would have to expose the secret to him. Hence, getting help with my rape trauma syndrome was out of the question.

Therefore, my childhood rape trauma defined how I raised my children; I was always aware of my surroundings, always on guard, on the lookout. I was constantly nervous, in the "fight or flight" mode; I learned that anything could happen to anyone, anywhere, and anytime. I realized as a child, I wasn't even safe hanging out in my front yard although this was a community where everyone knew one another. Consequently, if that environment was unsafe, then where does anyone feel secure?

I don't know how my poor sister managed psychologically after the rape experience she suffered that day. We have never spoken to each other about the effect it had on our lives. My sister is a strong person both physically and emotionally. However, any child who lived through what happened to us could never be the same person after that ordeal. That means, no matter how strong she is, she has to carry some lingering psychological issues. I imagine that she creates this strong persona from the outside while she suffers inside from the trauma of rape.

I know she is strong mentally, which will assist her in masking her pain. Hence, you would never know she had suffered any emotional issues by looking at her. So unless she would tell you of her lingering traumatic issues from that infamous day, you will never know of the impact it has on her life.

She was a young girl who experienced a vicious rape, so I am sure she had to suffer some trauma the way I suffered from the brutal rape. Rape Trauma Syndrome is colorless, it is odorless and invisible to the people around you. Even if you are very close to someone, you can never tell they are suffering (RTS). For these reasons, it usually hides in plain sight.

How I Will Tell My Children

I always wanted to tell my children about the rape my sister and I experienced when we were children. The problem was that I didn't know how to verbalize such a painful childhood experience to them. So essentially, I just never really told my children about it. I knew that it would cause some sadness for them to learn that I went through such an ordeal as a child. Thus, I decided that maybe it would be better if I kept the secret from everyone forever.

That decision was based on wanting to shield them from that sadness I felt years ago when the incident happened. My children are all adults now, so they will understand why I couldn't tell them about the rape when they were young kids. First of all, I had to feel ready to talk about something that caused me so much pain. Nonetheless, I am finally willing to speak about my childhood secret to everyone at this point in my life.

Now that I have written this book, naturally, my children will be the first ones to read it, and I will give them a heads up about the shocking content in this book before they proceed to read about it. I became bold enough to talk about what happened to me after the #MeToo movement started. It prompted me and gave me the courage I needed to move forward, so I decided to use this opportunity to talk about my very own #MeToo story.

I will warn them that this will not be an easy book for them to read and that it might be the most brutal book they have ever read in their life. Why? Because it has to do with some unpleasant news about their mom and aunt. I am the only one who can explain to them what exactly happened to us and how my rape trauma influenced the way I raised them.

When my now-adult children learn about the traumatic rape I experienced as a child, it will give them some perspective on why I was so protective of them when they were young children. They will realize that my rape memory initiated some of the decisions I made where they were concerned. I was not trying to be a difficult mama. I wanted to be the best protector for them, a protector that I needed to protect me on the day of the rape. My experience afforded me the awareness of some of the evil in the world. Therefore most of the decisions I made were because I was afraid for their safety.

My three children will be the first people outside of my sister and the two rapists to know what happened to us. I've lived with the big secret since the day it happened, and it is a part of my life that they had no idea about until now. I will invite them to ask me any question they have about that terrible day. It is an excellent feeling to know that I no longer have to keep that day a secret. And it is a freeing feeling for me to be able to share the secret with my children.

Now that they know the truth, this allows them to look back on some of my decisions involving them that frustrated and hurt them when they were children. For example, why I had a problem with playdates, sleepovers at friend's homes, sleepovers at day camps, and much more. My intention was not to hurt or control them; I did it out of my unconditional love for them. I didn't want them to have to live with the experience of rape for the rest of their lives like I had to. I wanted to spare them the pain of living with rape.

How I Freed Myself from the Secret

It is a very emotionally liberating experience for me to say I am finally free from the bondage of the secret. I no longer have a childhood secret holding me hostage. The embarrassment of my childhood rape left me feeling burdensome and inadequate. The feeling followed me into adulthood. It was not easy for me to eventually acknowledge and own what had happened to me. My first reaction was that I didn't have to admit it on a conscious level as long as I didn't speak about it. While subconsciously, it controlled my decisions and essentially my life.

By telling my story, I finally got the chance to have the freeing experience it afforded my spirit. When you can feel free from within, you emanate a certain glow from the inside out, and it is the best feeling in the world. Before writing this book, I thought that I had no other choice but to live an unauthentic secret life forever. One of my primary focuses in life was to ensure that the secret remains a secret forever. That conclusion was due to the shame of being raped; I had to ensure no one ever found out about what happened. I later realized that the secret I was protecting all these years was never my secret in the first place.

Although many prominent people had admitted to being sexually assaulted when they were children, one being the well-respected Oprah Winfrey, for some reason, I still didn't feel compelled to tell my story. Women come forward from time to time to speak about the unwanted sexual violation in their lives and how it affected them. And when they do, I would usually identify with what they had to say. However, I didn't feel like it was something I wanted to share at that time. I just wasn't ready to talk about what happened to me as a child. Considering I was not a celebrity, I thought no one would care about my story.

I never thought that I would be doing a positive service to my mental health by breaking the silent code. The stigma attached to rape, especially gang-rape, was so profound that it clogged my perception of what was in my best interest. All I could focus on was to carry the weight of ensuring that no one ever found out about the embarrassing dirty little secret.

I always wonder if there has ever been another case similar to ours. I am talking about a situation where two sisters got gang-raped together, basically side by side. If you know about a circumstance like ours, please share it with me. If it is still a secret and you are not ready to go public with your story, you can certainly remain anonymous. However, in the event that you feel comfortable enough to speak about it, you can tell me the outcome of your situation and how it has affected your life going forward. I am very interested in hearing about what happened.

That said, I don't have a precedent to compare to our horrific nightmare; our situation is rare as far as I know. I can't measure how my emotional state was affected against a similar case like ours where two sisters experience a rape together. Nonetheless, I am aware that all survivors will have a different perspective of the rape experience. However, shame is always a common denominator that links all victims/survivors of rape together.

After some courageous people decided that enough was enough, I wanted so badly to free myself from the secret I carried with me for years. I chose to capitalize on the brave women's synergy of the #MeToo movement and rid myself of my prison of shame. The energy at the moment supported me in telling my story. It gave me the strength to walk through the entrance after the movement kicked in the door. Finally, this started the well-deserved communication about rape and sexual misconduct at the hands of some selfish and cruel male perpetrators.

After I felt powerful enough emotionally, I developed the nerve to talk about my rape experience in detail. I always thought in my heart that it was unfair that my sister and I got raped, yet we were the ones who felt embarrassed for something we had no control over. A perfect example of blaming the victim of rape would be like blaming the people who were captured and turned into slaves for being caught.

The truth is that those people who were captured and enslaved had no control over their bodies. They were held captive and forced to work in some of the worst conditions possible without being paid. All the years of free labor affected the enslaved person's generational wealth to this day. Why would they willfully sabotage their own financial life?

The folks who called themselves "masters" of those enslaved individuals are the ones who should be embarrassed about their evil, inhumane actions. Their cruelty of not compensating the enslaved person for work performed has negatively affected the victims for many generations. In contrast, free work has benefited the "master's" generational wealth. That wealth has continued to flourish in their family to this day. Yet, society tries to paint the picture that the enslaved individuals should be embarrassed that they are poor.

The "slave masters" should be the ones to feel embarrassed that they were so vicious and had no empathy or any care for their fellow human beings. The people who were captured and forced to work without pay should not be ashamed of anything. They didn't do anything wrong; the perpetrators should be ashamed.

The same goes for the two rapists who held us against our will and raped us. They are the ones who should be embarrassed that they are going around holding young girls hostage and raping them in their homes. The culture was that the victims of sexual assault should be ashamed while the rapist walks around swaggering with heads held high.

Now that public opinion has shifted the rape shaming from the victims to the perpetrators, all I can say is that we finally got it right. The focus is where it should have always been, on the culprit. The rape shaming belongs to the sexual predators who committed those atrocious crimes. It is ridiculous that the victims of rape should ever get blamed and shamed for being rape; that is just victimizing them all over again.

This social shift has allowed so many of us to be free from the secret of being rape victims/survivors. We can now talk about our rape experience without being judged or scared of how others will perceive us.

For the first time since my sister and I got raped, I unveiled everything about the secret in this book. Plus, I get to use this opportunity to open the door for my sister and me to finally have that well-deserved conversation about that day. Since the gang-rape happened to us when we were young, we have never spoken to each other about it and how it has affected our lives. The shame and guilt associated with rape forced us to stay quiet.

I will give my sister a copy of this book before any reader peruses its content, and for the first time since the trauma, I will invite her to talk about what happened to us that day. I hope that she is ready for us to have a dialogue about it, and I'll finally learn how it has affected her emotionally.

I believe it is a long-overdue conversation for us to have with each other, and I am thrilled that we are both still alive to witness the day when one of us broke our silence. I hope that it will ease her mind when she and I talk about it, knowing it is okay now; we were only children when the rape occurred, and we didn't do anything wrong.

Even so, if my sister is still not ready to talk about the ordeal we suffered, I want her to know that it is okay as well. She can take as long as she wants and tell her story whenever and however she chooses, or not tell her story at all; it is her story and her choice. When it's all said and done, it remains her call. I will be the last person to force her to do anything she is not comfortable doing. I know first-hand the repercussion of being forced to participate without giving consent.

Writing This Book Helped Me

After I had suppressed my childhood rape trauma for most of my life, writing this book about my rape experience has become my therapy. I noticed that it has helped me stop suppressing my feelings about the rape trauma, and I discovered a way to co-exist with it as a part of my past.

I must admit that it wasn't an easy decision for me to write about the rape of my sister and me in detail. At first, my thoughts were, why should I put our secret out there for the world to see? But I also realized that once I started writing down what happened to us in-depth, I felt more and more liberated. I recognized that the more I recalled the rape memories that were suppressed and wrote them down, the freer and more empowered I felt. It didn't take long for me to recognize the benefit of writing down my feelings.

Consequently, writing down my experience freed me from the shameful intangible secret I took with me everywhere. I was no longer a prisoner of the shame that belonged to my perpetrators. I held the rape shame for them for too long; it was not mine to keep any longer.

Another thing that was therapeutic for me was writing down several questions I wanted to ask both rapists. I looked at it as though I finally got a chance to ask them some critical questions, questions that had haunted me for years. I always wanted to know the answers to some of the confusion I felt. Despite the fact that I may never get these answers, I am still grateful for my journey to freedom.

Writing down my questions allowed me to visualize both of them with their heads bowed down in shame. The rape shame was finally off my shoulders and placed on both rapists, exactly where it belonged. It was not my shame to carry any further because it was never my shame in the first place. I hope that this book will be seen by the two rapists one of these days. And hopefully, they will be able to answer some of these questions for themselves.

In any case, I don't think I need to hear what they have to say at this point; I am good knowing that I got to ask my questions in writing. Both rapists can read the questions and answer them for their conscience, if they have any. It is going to have to be between them and Karma. According to The Law of Karma, every action has an equal and opposite reaction. If you do good deeds, you will receive good results, and if you do bad things, you are creating bad karmas for yourself. Whatever you sow, you will reap, so at this point, it's up to their God to conclude an outcome for them. The fact is you must be careful of the energy you put out into the world because it has a ripple effect.

A part of my decision to write this book was so that my children could know about the other part of my childhood experience that I've never disclosed to them. I've never revealed the rape I experienced because of the stigma attached to that part of my life. I know now that the shame I carried with me all these years belongs to the two rapists. It is a liberating feeling for me not to take their guilt with me any longer.

I also use this opportunity to let both rapists know how their selfish and controlling actions changed the course of my life, and that it had a significant effect on how I raised my children. I hope to educate rapists worldwide about how devastating their choices are when choosing to use sexual assault of any type to impose control over someone else.

Sexual predators should be aware that their acts of sexual misconduct are demoralizing to the individuals they are victimizing. When a sex predator decides to commit rape, that cruel and selfish decision doesn't necessarily stop there. It can essentially continue to live on in the victim's next generation. The thoughtless and careless decisions the predators make can negatively affect the victim's second and third generations. Studies show that a victim of rape will parent their children differently. Those children will also parent their children from that same rape experience that they have learned from the rape survivor who raised them.

Writing down what happened to me has helped me cope emotionally and psychologically. It allowed me to go back to that awful day and retrieve all the suppressed memories in detail; these are memories that were lodged deep inside my subconscious mind. The memories were blocking my energy from flowing correctly and were making me physically sick. Recording the evil in writing has forced me to face the demons that kept me locked in scared mode all these years. The secret forced me to live my life in fear of having it revealed. Now, I'm telling the world the secret, and I'm doing it MY way.

It was a relief for me, and as I recalled the memories and wrote them down, I realized that the memories of that infamous day just started to flow like raindrops. The secret that was in my subconscious mind all these years was ready to be told. It didn't want to stay in hiding any longer; that is the reason my spirit finally felt free.

When someone suffers these traumas, they usually never go away totally; it becomes a staple in the subconscious mind. The subconscious mind is like a tape player, it records information and plays them back repeatedly. When individuals suffer from such rape traumas, they are always on the lookout for the "what-ifs" to happen. Those who experienced rape will always prepare themselves psychologically in that fight or flight mode. In doing this, they would be ready either way if something were to happen.

The victim of rape can readily recall, at will, the vicious memories of the incident. Those memories can show up at anytime and anywhere, and the fight or flight sensations are an obvious trigger for the rape anxiety to return.

For someone who suffers from Rape Trauma Syndrome, I can guarantee you that the suppressed memories can easily be a trigger, and can cause the victim to live in fear. The unfortunate thing is that this kind of assault will never go away completely. Personally, I just pretty much learned to cope with it the best way I could, despite my anxiety.

Due to the stigma attached to rape, some survivors are afraid of even using the word rape. Several rape victims/survivors are scared to say they got raped. The reason for that is because they are in denial about it. The last thing some rape survivors want to do is acknowledge that they got violated in that way. They are stuck in denial that the rape happened.

If you are a survivor of rape or if you are unsure if it was rape or not, the moment you have to wonder about consent, then there is a problem. If you are blaming yourself for the rape, thinking that maybe it was something you did that provoked the action of the abuser, you have to remember that consent is not ambiguous. The English word yes is evident and easy to understand.

Suppose you are confused about what took place and you don't want to use the word rape, just in case you might be wrong. You must understand that if a sexual act happened to you and is frustrating you as to what exactly it was or what transpired, you may need to take a closer look at the situation. And if you were a child when it happened, there is no other way about it; you got raped.

The law clearly states that children cannot give sexual consent. So you need to put this book down and go and tell somebody right now. Give them this book to read, and it will open the conversation about sexual assault/rape. In any case, the fear of humiliation if you use the correct terms (rape) only helps the perpetrators stay safe. It also keeps the victims in a psychological prison for a long time.

I know that the fear of being seen by others as damaged goods is devastating, and if you get gang-raped, the stigma is even worse. Furthermore, the shame attached to the label of being viewed as a "bad girl" is painful. This label meant a promiscuous girl who runs around with many different men. The sad reality is that a rape victim can sometimes become promiscuous because of having low self-esteem due to being sexually violated.

That is especially true if the girl was traumatized by rape at a very young age. It is crucial to know that the stigma of rape is not only for girls. No, the bias goes across the board to both genders; the shame of being disrespected by sexual assault or rape can happen to both males and females. It can cause the victims to self-destruct, mainly because the rape robbed them of their self-respect. The act destroys the individual's self-worth; it causes them to feel less than their identity.

Rape victims/survivors who are still in denial about sexual assault, I hope you can feel some comfort in knowing that as soon as you feel comfortable calling the act that happened to you by its actual name – rape (if that is what happened) -you will feel liberated, and it will help you to feel better about yourself.

Some rape survivors may feel that if they said the word rape out loud, they admit that the rape happened to them. And if the secret is out, they might be seen as damaged goods and all the other negative words associated with women who fall victim to rape.

Some victims/survivors may feel that if they stay quiet and don't say anything about the rape, it will disappear from their psyche. And they will never have to think about it ever again. They believe that not speaking about it will help them pretend the rape didn't happen.

If that is what you think, well, let me tell you that I tried doing that, and it didn't help me. Instead, it hitched itself deep in my subconscious mind. It influenced many of the life decisions I made from that hiding spot, including my parenting decisions. So, don't ever think that by you not saying the word "rape", you can simply move on with your life and forget that it happened. I can tell you that it's not so simple. You will not be able to freely allow it to be a part of your life until you can acknowledge that the rape happened.

Take it from me when I tell you that you should face the sexual violation you suffered head-on and admit that it occurred as a part of your healing. Know that if you didn't consent to having sex with someone, if you opposed the act, yet it happened without your permission, then you were raped. If this happened to you, there are no two ways about it; you got raped. You must first acknowledge that it happened before you can move forward.

You have to understand that this experience will be with you for the rest of your life; like it or not, your life has changed in an instant the day the rape transpired. Admit to yourself that an unwanted sexual assault took place. You may never be able to strip away the shame and guilt attached to sexual assault and rape in the world, but if you don't come to terms with the cause of your deep-seated pain, then you will never be able to find a way for you and that horrible experience to co-exist.

The moment you can speak freely about it, without any shame and guilt, that is when you will know for sure that it's all coming together, and you are recovering. And only you can make that happen; you have to be open and ready for the healing to take place within you.

Although I may have accepted the experience as a part of my journey on this earth school where I came to learn and grow, I can't say that it's still not there in my subconscious mind. I will never be able to rid myself of the memory of what those two evil rapists did to us. And it will still hurt me emotionally whenever any situation triggers it. However, I used writing to rid myself of its shame and its guilt. I placed those emotions on both rapists where they belong.

Moving forward, I don't feel the guilt and shame about being raped anymore. That's because I have accepted it as a part of my story, and I know where the shame and guilt belong. I know that I could not have done anything as a child to invite two adult rapists to gang-rape me. It was not my fault; it was that of the predators, who went around victimizing children by raping them.

Both rapists are the ones who made that horrible decision to hurt us that day, and the decision they made had nothing to do with me or my sister. They decided to steal our innocence and left us with this awful rape experience that we have to live with for the rest of our lives. Yes, I agree that the shame belongs somewhere, but it doesn't belong to the victims. It's the predator's shame. They ought to be ashamed of themselves for choosing the act of rape as a weapon against females and males. I can't even fathom the thought of how someone could be so cruel, especially to children.

I can only hope that there is something in this book that can help someone out there to cope with an unwanted sexual experience. I am happy to share with you that writing about my rape experience has helped me tremendously. So, writing down what you would like to say to the predators does wonder for your mental health. I find that it worked for me emotionally by giving me peace and clarity.

Don't get me wrong, I am not here to tell you that what works for me will also work for you because everyone has a different experience. And depending on your experience, you may need to use another tool to cope with your life's obstacles. Nevertheless, everything is worth a try, and in the long run you are the one who will have to save yourself. I can only show you one way that can help you to protect your sanity. But when all is said and done, you will be the one who will have to defend yourself by coming to terms with your rape trauma memories.

I can only tell you that I know for sure that you will have to acknowledge what happened to you before you can be free of the secret. For example, suppose rape is a part of your story, you will have to practice saying the word "rape" enough times until it flows freely without the feeling of shame attached to you getting raped.

I know for sure that writing the word rape enough times will liberate you, which is a freeing feeling. Therefore, I can attest that it worked for me. As soon as I decided to acknowledge that the rape happened to me, I could use the word rape and call both rapists for what they were - "rapists". That was when my recovery started. After I did that, I finally felt liberated and free of the shame and stigma attached to survivors of rape.

I realized that the moment I changed the way I perceived the rape, I clearly saw where the shame belonged. I started to feel free, and I slowly became much more open to talk about my experience. When I said I changed how I looked at the rape, I started to look at my shame logically. That's why I used the slave analogy to show the difference in perception. When you perceive the narrative differently, you usually get a different result. It is like what Wayne Dyer said, "When you change the way you look at things, the things you look at change."

After examining my shame and the reason I was ashamed, I realized that I had no control to hinder it from happening; I tried to stop it, but I failed. It had nothing to do with me and everything to do with the two rapists who decided to rape children. That is the same way slavery had everything to do with the evil slave "masters" who stole other humans from their homeland and worked them to the bones against their will.

I am hopeful that the shame associated with slave "masters" will be the same shame directed to the sex predators. The enslavement robbed those humans of their dignity and caused them to lose their self-respect. Nowadays, out of embarrassment, the beneficiary of the slave trade will never admit their generational wealth is coming from their ancestor's slave trade business. A certain stigma is associated with the slave trade generational wealth passed down from the greedy slave "masters."

The slave "masters" wanted to show how powerful they were; they wanted to build generational wealth. The free labor afforded them that luxury and it helped them to create their wealth faster. The evil rapists wanted to show the power they had over two young girls.

How could slavery have anything to do with the people it enslaved? Likewise, how could the rape of my sister and I have anything to do with us? We were not even at the age to give consent because we were children when it happened. We would never invite them into our home to rape us. They decided on their own that day to drag us from our front yard into our house where we were humiliated and brutally raped by two adult rapists.

When I wrote about my rape experience, I found that the step-by-step approach I used allowed me to strip away the shame I carried all these years, one layer at a time. And the more I wrote the word rape, the more I could use it shamelessly. So writing has helped me live with the rape situation as a part of my life experience. I am pleased that I can openly admit that I got raped as a child without having the feeling of embarrassment.

I should also mention that you have to be ready emotionally and psychologically to talk openly about your rape experience. I used the strength of all the people who used #MeToo to talk about their rape and unwanted sexual demons. It helped me to develop the courage to talk about being one of the #MeToo individuals.

I noticed that the more I started to use the word rape, the more I felt a sense of empowerment, bit by bit. Let's face it, my sister and I were traumatized that day. As I mentioned before, we didn't invite this experience into our lives. But since it became a part of our life, we had to live with our reality.

If you are still blaming yourself and feeling scared and ashamed of a rape you endured, stop blaming yourself for something you had no control over. It's not your fault; you were molested or raped. How can you be blamed for not having the physical strength to fight off a heartless predator? It's not your fault; there was nothing you could do to prevent it from happening; you didn't do anything wrong.

When you remain silent about the rape, you will indirectly help protect the perpetrators. Your silence gives them power and assists them to continue looking for their next victim. I'm sorry to say, but your silence will not help you in any way. Use whatever it takes to build up your emotional strength to take your power back from the predator.

The predator is the weak one who makes sure to prey on girls or boys who are no match for themselves physically. You are the strong one who lived through that ordeal and continues to rise. Repeat these three words several times every day: I am strong!

You may be able to use some of the information here to help free yourself from the shame of the unwanted sexual assault that attaches itself to you. But, for you to do so, your acknowledgment of the rape is your first step; then, the healing will come.

In this book, you may have noticed that I did not, for once, call the predators anything but rapists and predators. The reason for that is because I didn't want to humanize them. I have to call them precisely what they were. I had to remember them for how cruel and heartless they were to us that day. There was nothing about their treatment towards us that could even come remotely close for me to define them as human.

I recalled them being very uncaring and cruel to us. To fully come to grips with my story, I have to use any method to help me with my mental health. And if it means that I have to get angry and see them as the lowest scum of the earth for robbing me of a life without a rape experience, I'm sorry, but that is what I had to do to speak about the effect their wrong decision had on my life.

Also, I wanted to remember them in their inhumane natural habitat. This approach helped me heal when it comes to getting rid of my shame and guilt. My perception of the two rapists is that they are bullies. The more I refer to them as rapists or predators, the more I feel stronger and bolder to talk about what they did to us without any shame.

The feeling of disrespect and violation beyond your control might still be there for a while. But keep your focus on replacing that with knowing that the shame is on the sexual abuser, that it has nothing to do with you. Every time you feel the shame and guilt trigger nudging at you as it tries to come into your consciousness, replace it by putting the shame back where it belongs, on the rapist. The humiliation belongs to the predators.

The humiliation is always on the sexual predators that go around preying on others. I hope some of this information can help someone out there suffering from Rape Trauma Syndrome. The moment I finally faced the rape experience head-on and spoke about my reality in detail, it took away my shame and fear. I was able to place those emotions with the rapist finally and that is where they always belong. This approach has helped me to rid myself of the shame and guilt I carried around for years. I hope this can inspire you to do whatever it takes to overcome the shame you are carrying around for your sexual abuser; it is their shame, it's not yours.

To recap, writing this book helped me by giving me a safe place where I could talk about my experience in detail without shame. Speaking about my experience helped free me from the secret I carried around with me for many years. When I called the rape action rape instead of sexual assault, it was very liberating.

All being well, this can help to inspire other sufferers to free themselves by talking about the unpleasant rape secret that they are still carrying for the rapist.

Ask yourself, why are you keeping the secret that belongs to the rapist? It's not your secret to keep forever; it has absolutely nothing to do with you. When you burden yourself by hiding the rape that happened to you, you are protecting the rapist. It's time to stop and focus on what's best for you; "Time's up."

I lived with a rape experience that was always front and center in my life; it influenced many of my life decisions. Writing helped me immensely to rid myself of the shame associated with rape. I found that this book helped me to finally get a chance to revisit the worst day of my life. I've never really looked back on that day in its entirety until now. Being able to review the pain of that day wasn't easy for me to do, but one of the positive things about it is that I was finally able to say the word "rape."

In short, it was worth revisiting. I never really went back to that hard place emotionally since I became an adult, and that's because it was a harrowing experience for me to relive. The writing has forced me to go back to that scary place to collect the painful details of what happened to us that day.

To elaborate on the rape that happened to my sister and me, I frequently mentioned the word rape. I'm pleased to declare that doing so has helped me gradually strip away the shame and guilt I carried around for decades. I didn't want to sugar-coat the act by calling it words like sexual assault or sexual misconduct.

I didn't use those words to explain what happened to us because they are too vague and confusing. And they left the reader with many questions as to what exactly happened. When I said we got gang-raped, it's not confusing to the reader about the depth of the trauma we experienced.

I used the words sexual assault and sexual misconduct a few times in writing this book, but I feel that it doesn't explain what I experienced. It is my reality, and my experience was that I suffered a traumatic rape experience. For me, calling the act anything but rape would minimize the level of what we lived through that day. I had to watch my sister as she got raped, and then it was my turn to be raped by both rapists. We were both gang-raped in our own home. The experience I went through was not a sexual assault – not in my mind, it wasn't; we were both raped.

Forgive me if it makes you feel uncomfortable; I am sorry. If you are uncomfortable hearing about the words I used to describe what happened to us, then think about what two young girls went through on that dreadful day together. It took me a very long time to build up the courage to talk about what happened in our home that day. But now, I finally have the nerve to free myself from the prison of secrecy and shame. I can tell you that the last thing I want to do is use words that I feel will reduce what we experienced, only so that someone else can feel comfortable.

After I witnessed my sister brutally tortured by rape, it was my turn to face the same fate as she did. It was her turn to watch and listen to me suffering like I had to watch and listen to her suffering. The immeasurable trauma I suffered after the horrific experience left me emotionally wounded for many years. So now that I finally feel comfortable talking about it, I choose to use the words I feel appropriate to describe what happened to us.

I believe the last thing that I should do is to use the term "sexually assaulted" instead of "rape." The purpose of this book is not to make other people feel comfortable. My goal is to be able to free myself from the rape shame. Therefore, at this moment, I want to do what is best for me, and the label of sexual assault is not the suffering I felt. And it wasn't the suffering I continued to endure psychologically for many years afterward.

Writing this book gave me a platform to speak as though I was speaking directly to both rapists. I got to ask the questions that plagued me for many years. Even if I never get them to answer why two adult rapists would feel the need to gang-rape two children in their home, just by me getting the chance to potentially let both rapists know that I have shifted the shame from my sister and myself, I have placed it in its rightful place with them where it belongs.

When you consider everything, there is no way the shame could have been with two young girls who were hanging out in our front yard. We didn't do anything to either of them, and we didn't invite two rapists into our home to be traumatized and gang-raped. Why were we ever made to be ashamed of what they did to us in the first place? I suppose I will never know the answer to that program we got as humans. Thankfully we are trying to correct the wrong in our lifetime.

I traded my shame to both rapists for their freedom. Once and for all, I finally know what it feels like to be free of their secret that burdened me for years. What they did to us was a criminal offense as stipulated by the law of the land. Both of them committed two counts of statutory rape, two counts of unlawful restrictions and kidnapping for holding us against our will, and so many other charges. And spiritually, they both went against everything that the soul stands for; one being do unto others as you would like them to do unto you. I agree that we all have free will, but you should never use your free will to hurt others.

Thank You Ladies and Gentlemen

I am thankful to the super great ladies and some stand-up men for finally having the courage to support what was right and call out the sexual predators for who they were. It is tough to imagine that a few men among us can be so disrespectful to women. And to know that those same men have women in their lives, they all have mothers, sisters, daughters, aunts, and cousins who are females, saddened a part of me.

Let me remind the small percentage of men who disrespect women that you are a part of us. We are your moms and your family; a woman will always stand by your side and protect you no matter what; by nature, that's what we do. We love and need you much more than you think, and for the real men who see us as equals and not as prey, thanks for your courage and for having our backs. Those women who afforded me the courage to speak about my rape experience without feeling embarrassed, I appreciate you.

Why should I be forced to feel ashamed for something I couldn't control? The whole notion surrounding that is insane. It has never been deemed unsafe in our district for us to hang out in our front yard. Living in a warm climate, people were usually outside in their yards, so it was not an unusual occurrence. It was something everyone did without any issues.

People living on the island will only go inside the house to eat or sleep; other than that, everyone is usually outside. Not to mention the fact that we were living in the country. On the island, it is summer weather all year round. This means that as soon as we were up in the mornings, we would go outdoors to feed the chickens and do other outdoor chores. If the kids don't hang out outside the house like we did when we were children, it would be because of all the electronic gadgets available to them these days. So if there are some changes, I still don't think it would be that much of a difference.

I'm sure that the youngsters can still hang out in their front yards without having to worry about being raped. This is especially true when you live in the country as I did where everyone knows everyone else. Our situation was not a common occurrence that I was aware of in our community, where young girls were dragged into their houses from outside and raped in the middle of the day. I don't know of any other situation in our district that was similar to our gang-bang experience. Then again, the girls would more or less keep it quiet out of shame. For the most part, living in the country was supposed to be safer than living in the big city.

If a stranger were to show up in our community, the community would immediately inquire about who the individual was. They would ask around to see if that new person was related to anyone they knew. And, sure enough, we would usually get to the bottom of it very quickly.

Usually, when the community puts out its inquiry about the new person, I can assure you that we would know who the stranger was by the end of the day. When living in the big cities such as Kingston, it would be much different in terms of identifying people and immediately knowing their background as you are more likely to see strangers daily. On the other hand, the two rapists who raped us were no strangers to us; they were two of our community members.

Raising Compassionate Men Can Teach Empathy

Here are my thoughts on raising our youths, what if we nurture our boys to be more compassionate? Would that help those compassionate boys to grow up and become kind individuals? I wonder if that would enable the small percentage of men who rape and disrespect women to understand and respect girls' and women's feelings.

Some parents of boys believe that raising their sons to be rugged and tough is essential. They don't emphasize encouraging them to be vulnerable and empathetic with others, especially women. Suppose there was a way to encourage boys to be more caring towards girls instead of seeing girls and women as sexual objects and prey? If they had all those qualities, they would be a great addition to society. The two rapists who raped us had no compassion for us.

Let us look at some ways that men and women play similar roles to where they differ. We know that men and women have no problems when choosing the same career path most of the time. Here are a few examples of some professions that both men and women hold momentarily:

1. Police officers
2. Firefighters
3. Doctors
4. Lawyers
5. Entrepreneurs
6. Teachers
7. Marketers
8. Sales
9. Daycare workers
10. Nurses

Both sexes share so many more careers; these are only to name a few.

What if we start with the dads mentoring their young sons to develop their sensitive and compassionate side? That means they would have to ignore the negative stereotypes that boys have to be masculine and rugged. When we look at most statistics so far, we are doing great with the girls, but there are still specific careers that men are wary of pursuing.

Dr. Ted Zeff wrote an article in which he said that "Women now make up close to half the enrollment in United States law and medical schools, up from less than twenty-five percent a few decades ago." Dr. Zeff said, "Men continue to shun nursing as a career; only about eight percent of registered nurses are male."

That is an example of what I am talking about: why are young men afraid of embarking on a nursing career? The article spoke to how our sons feel that they will be perceived by their peers or sometimes by their parents in a certain light when they consider pursuing a nursing career.

Years ago, I wanted to go into the trucking career (you heard me correctly, I was going to drive the big rig trucks). I always admired the few AZ female drivers when they would pull up their big trucks at one of their delivery stops and jump out of that monster truck to do the delivery.

It was amazing when I saw the small woman jump out of the driver's side of that massive beast of a truck that she controls on the road. You can't imagine how passionate I still feel when I talk about it. Nonetheless, I promise I won't bore you by going on about it, but I still think it is darn cool to see a woman pushing down a big rig truck on the highway.

That said, let me tell you what happened to my dream. I fell into the stereotype that women should not be truck drivers. I registered for college, and a friend of mine asked me what I was going to study. When I told her I had a passion for the trucking industry, she laughed at me. I then changed my major to business, and she didn't laugh when I went into this program. She was exposed to that stereotype constructed in her environment which influenced women to feel as if they should not be truck drivers. I succumbed to her judgment, believed, and gave up on my dream.

I suppose the environment I grew up in was different from that of most people. After all, how many people get to be raised by a single dad? I grew up with a dad who didn't put any limits on us, and that was why I could picture myself driving a big rig truck. I didn't have any reservations about it until my friend started to laugh at me. I thought that if she was laughing it must mean that it's not an admirable profession for a woman.

That said, I know firsthand how influential peer pressure can be. After my friend laughed, I didn't bother to pursue that dream because I was affected by her perception of the world. I instead went into the Business program where I studied Business Administration and majored in Human Resources. We had many male students in my classes at the time, but most of the students in my business classes were females.

According to authors Dan Kindlon and Michael Thompson, "Dads treat their daughters differently than their sons." Research has shown that fathers treat their infant daughters more gently than they do baby boys. I'm not saying that this is the issue that caused some men to feel the need to control women. I'm just looking for similarities and differences in the way we raise our boys and girls, and how that environment influences the way they perceive the world.

The authors said, "As the children grow up, fathers tend to show their sons less physical affection, correct them more often, and play more competitively with them." This example of the dads' behavior is that he teaches the boys to be rough, which is fine, but there has to be a balance. Both genders need to grow up with love and affection. They should be encouraged to behave in a caring and compassionate manner.

What if we start by having girls and boys doing the same household chores just like men and women can have the same profession? Not only should we have gender-neutral duties, but they should also be encouraged to help each other with their chores. Learning to help one another will encourage the kids to build kindness and empathy for each other.

Some examples of gender-neutral chores are:

1. The boys do the dishes, and the girls do the dishes.
2. The boys mow the lawn, the girls mow the lawn.
3. The boys do the laundry, and the girls can do the laundry.
4. The boys can help with the grocery, and the girls can help with the grocery.
5. The boys help with meal preparation, and the girls help with meal preparation.
6. The boys help to shovel the snow, the girls help to shovel the snow
7. The boys help care for the younger siblings, and the girls help care for the younger siblings.
8. The boys take care of the animals, the girls take care of the animals.

When your children realize that jobs and careers are genderless, this will instill in them that they are on an equal playing field. As long as they are equal and there is no hierarchy between genders, they will learn to respect each other, and everything else will fall into place. When this happens, it means that we have raised our boys to be strong, compassionate males and raised our girls to be strong, compassionate females.

The Dali Lama said, "It takes a strong man to be a compassionate man." When our children are raised and nurtured as solid and compassionate people, we are more likely to have empathetic men. And we will be able to eliminate a wide variety of issues that plague us for generations—for example, sexual assault, harassment of all kinds, and rape.

Love Teaches Compassion:

1. The boys get hugs from mom and dad, the girls get hugs from mom and dad.
2. The boys get reassurance that they are loved, the girls get reassurance that they are loved.
3. Boys are allowed to get emotional and cry without being criticized that they should be tough. As well, girls are allowed to get emotional and cry.
4. Boys get to help grandma and grandpa shovel the snow and cut the lawn, girls get to help grandma and grandpa shovel the snow and mow the lawn.

It is essential to try and make a conscious decision not to separate chores for your sons and daughters based on gender from an early age. I am an example that genderless duties can be beneficial to both girls and boys. I grew up without gender-based chores and genderless careers. That is why I didn't see a truck driving profession to be a man's job. We were fortunate to be raised as children instead of as a girl child or a boy child. We didn't even play gender-based sports; we played every type of sport.

There are many areas of my life where my upbringing came in very handy. One of those times was when my husband left our family and I instantly got thrown into the single-mom role with three small children. Eventually, all the duties and responsibilities my ex-husband and I shared were now my duties.

Accordingly, I had no option but to pick up the torch and lead my little angels into the future as the head of the household. I was now in charge of everything my husband used to do in our home. Although my obligations instantly doubled, the good news was that I knew how to do everything. I even had a toolbox with my tools just in case I needed them. Let's say I knew how to do many things such as painting our house, cutting the lawn, and cleaning the snow.

These are some of the reasons you should have gender-neutral duties. Teach your boys and girls how to do everything; it will help them be well-rounded, and if life knocks them down, they will be able to get up, dust themselves off and continue onward. Teach your children kindness, it helps to build inner strength, and that strength will increase empathy. When your child is empathetic, they will grow up to be compassionate and caring adults. Compassion breeds love and respect, and when you respect others, you are less likely to want to do anything to hurt them.

When we teach our boys compassion from a very young age, it will let them know that compassion doesn't mean that they are weak. It means they are strong men who are not afraid to be vulnerable. Vulnerability means that your boys are strong human beings with lots of emotions, and it opens the door for communication. They won't feel scared of being ridiculed to open up and speak about what's bothering them.

Essentially, those boys will grow up to become fathers. Those new fathers will raise their children and teach them that being vulnerable doesn't mean they are weak. Ultimately, we will break the cycle that men are weak if they show their emotional side.

Teach Random Acts of Kindness - Teach Compassion

Parents should try to teach kindness by example to their children as empathy formulates compassion. When people are kind, they are less than likely to hurt others. Children tend to emulate their parents so let them see you helping out other less fortunate people than yourself.

If you are assisting an elderly neighbor with yard work or helping someone bring groceries inside out of the cold, invite your children to get involved. These acts of kindness will enable the next generation of people to develop compassion by showing love and kindness.

Having compassion can lead to increased happiness and freedom from gender stereotypes. It can build a better overall relationship with others; kindness gives rise to gratitude, joy, and happiness. Don't get me wrong. I am not saying that this way is the answer for every person. However, one way we can pass on empathy to the next generation is to lead by example. We can start by teaching them how to show love and compassion to others.

All of us should try as much as we can to use love and empathy to teach compassion. The two rapists, who raped my sister and me, came from families that seemed very normal from the outside. But I don't know what was going on inside of their homes.

The first rapist was from a pretty decent family. He had an older sister who was a teacher; he was the middle child and his younger brother was a very decent, educated man who was certainly not a rapist.

As I mentioned before, I was not living in their home so I don't know about his nurturing. I am well aware that children raised in the same household may have different nurturing experiences from their siblings growing up. Every child is different and has different needs and will see the world and people through a different lens from their siblings. All siblings have their perceptions of how they grew up, and it doesn't make them good or bad people; we all perceive the world differently.

Most parents do the best they can with the tools they have at the time. But there is a moral responsibility that all humans should be taught respect and kindness, is necessary no matter what the conditions are. It has to be recognized that we must try and break that cycle of cruelty and disrespect towards one another. All I know is that those rapists had no respect or compassion for us.

The first rapist's brother was a completely different person from him; they were like night and day. We once had a community youth club in our district and his brother was the president of this youth club. I knew his brother very well. He was a decent and well-respected individual in our community and he would never rape anyone.

The second rapist was from a decent family as well, and he was from a huge family; ironically, he had many sisters. Yet again, I do not know how the nurturing was at his home, so I can't speak on that. I can only tell you what I know for sure about him. I know that he was a rapist, and I know that he had no respect or compassion for neither my sister nor me. I can say this because he was the one who restrained me until his friend was ready to rape me.

He then went on to rape my sister, and then he took turns to rape me after his friend raped me. They were both very cruel and disrespectful to us; they had hearts that were as cold as ice. And they couldn't care less about us; we were treated by them as if we were nothing.

In an article in Greater Good Magazine written by Kozo Hattori, the article's headline was, "What does it take to foster compassion in men?" To find out the answer to his question, Kozo Hattori interviewed scientific and spiritual experts. He said, "All of the compassionate men I interviewed, they all broke out of the *'act-like-a-man'* box." They didn't want to live the rest of their lives and not show vulnerability; they will look weak if they do. Therefore they decided to leave that paradigm behind. They changed how they looked at things, and the things they looked at changed - (Dr. Wayne Dyer).

Dr. Rick Hanson, the author of Hardwiring Happiness, said compassion makes an individual more courageous because compassion strengthens the heart. He said he realized that he was too left-brained, so he made a conscious effort at a certain point to reconnect with his intuitive, emotional side. Things are changing for the best; men are starting to realize that compassion is a strength, not a weakness. It is never too late to evaluate yourself and consciously change for the better.

When Thich Nhat Hanh, the Zen Buddhist Monk, was asked by a writer, "How could we make compassion more attractive to men?" He answered, "There must be a fundamental misunderstanding about the nature of compassion because compassion is very powerful; compassion protects us more than guns, bombs, and money."

Most men don't want to teach compassion to their sons or show their caring side because they are afraid of being viewed as weak instead of empathetic and strong. But in reality, it is quite on the contrary; it takes a strong man to be a compassionate man. And a strong empathetic man can never be a rapist because they can easily put themselves in another person's shoes.

Therefore, by teaching your sons to be compassionate, you teach them to be strong human beings. If a boy learns to get in touch with his feminine side from an early age, it will solve many of our society's problems today. Issues such as being disrespectful to women, sexual assaults, and otherwise, could probably be eliminated.

I grew up with four sisters and one brother, our single dad raised us and he had never treated any of us differently based on our gender. Our father's expectations for his girls were no different from his expectations for his son; we've never had girl chores separate from boy chores in our household. Nevertheless, we were aware that many kids in our neighborhood had different duties allotted to them based on their gender.

We all respected one another in our home as humans; my father had never told my brother to do certain chores because he is a man. Neither has he told him to man-up, or be a real man. We were lucky that we never had to deal with that type of upbringing. Thank goodness, that type of communication was never a part of our household's vocabulary as children. Now that we are adults, I've never heard of any women or girls being disrespected sexually by my brother.

Random acts of kindness reveal that when you raise a compassionate son, he is more than likely to stand up for a child at school whom other children are bullying. Your child is more likely to accompany that child to report the incident to the teacher. Those qualities show the strength of an empathetic child who will grow up to be an empathetic adult.

It takes solid and compassionate parents to raise compassionate children. I cannot say this enough that neither of the two rapists we encountered that day had any compassion for us. If their parents had raised them to be empathetic, loving, and compassionate, it would have stayed with them into adulthood. The love in those adults would prevent them from doing anything to hurt another person. Accordingly, it would be less likely for them to commit a rape or any unwanted sexual act against others.

I am not saying that teaching compassion is the answer to solving all sexual assault problems. Sometimes, mental issues drive people to commit various crimes, and some of those crimes include rape. But what I am saying is that we can use compassion and love to teach empathy, and with empathy comes love, and love is the answer to kindness. Kindness can be a simple way of controlling violence to some extent. Nevertheless, it is not the only solution as crime and violence stems from many factors.

When you feel for another person on an empathetic level, you are less likely to hurt that person. We can't just leave our children to learn these skills on their own, we have to teach love by example, and we have to start teaching love from the day they are born. Suppose you were never exposed to empathy yourself, you would certainly lack the ability to truly care for someone. By all means, it is in the best interest of your children when you practice being kind.

In Gary Zukav's book The Seat of The Soul, he said, "Without awareness of our feelings we cannot experience compassion, how can we share the suffering and joy of others if we cannot experience our own." It is essential to teach empathy to your children, and the best way to teach is by example.

The rape experience we suffered by the two rapists revealed that they had no love in their hearts. The lack of love for us is the reason they could have made such a horrible decision to hurt us the way they did. Both of them treated us very inhumanely and without any feeling of sympathy for us. It is essential to teach children to be respectful to others; teach them that vulnerability is not a weakness but it shows strength.

I learned from my childhood rape experience that anything can happen to anyone, anywhere, and that some people are heartless. I can tell you now that my pain is one of my stories; it doesn't define who I am as a person. In this book, I talked about my pain, and I told you about my reality. I spoke about how I overcame the secret and how I returned it to its rightful place.

I know that before I could come to grips with what happened to me, I would first have to accept that it occurred, and I have done that. I know that I will have to coexist with the rape experience as part of my life journey.

I have since learned to deal with my past, and I carry no adverse feelings towards the predators. I can assure you that I didn't do it for them; I did it to help myself on my journey. It helped me free myself from the resentment and hate that can eat one alive. Now that I have returned the shame, I have since moved forward into the next chapter of my life.

My suggestion to parents everywhere is for you to let your children know that the door is always wide open for them to speak to you about everything and anything. So even if they share with you a silly story that happened at school, show them that you are interested in the story by engaging in the conversation and probing. When you listen with interest to what your children have to share, it will build communication and trust in your relationship with them. Good luck and blessings to you all.

www.ingramcontent.com/pod-product-compliance
Lightning Source LLC
Chambersburg PA
CBHW070907080526
44589CB00013B/1204